Praise for *"Where's my shoes?"*

"A powerful encapsulation of what one can hope to get by spending several years in a lively support group! Brenda brings a priceless gift to those who doubt their capabilities or feel alone in the undertaking. Her story is animated and endearingly hopeful in the midst of uncertainty and disappointments.

Brenda's empowering and compassionate message, from one caregiver to the multitudes she mentors, is like a song that stays with you for a very long time."

Jill Wilson, MS
Geriatric Services Manager,
South Region Aurora Health Care

"It cannot be denied that *Where's My Shoes?* is a love story. On the surface it tells the true story in real time, as Brenda faces reality and makes hard, yet informed decisions. But between the lines, it's about the youngest daughter taking responsibility for family affairs and the care of her beloved father."

Mark Warner
Co-founder: www.alzstore.com
Author, *The Complete Guide to Alzheimer's-Proofing Your Home*

"Brenda has chronicled each step of the caregiver's journey with compassion, humor, and truth. A must read for professionals working with older adults and for all families affected by Alzheimer's disease and related dementias."

Kathleen Hairston
Area Program Manager
Sunrise Senior Living

NEWLY REVISED AND EXPANDED SECOND EDITION

"WHERE's mySHOES?"

My Father's Walk through Alzheimer's

The author openly reveals details about
caring for one with dementia.

BRENDA AVADIAN, MA

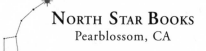

NORTH STAR BOOKS
Pearblossom, CA

Aricept® is a registered trademark of Pfizer and Eisai.
Safe Return™ is a trademark of the Alzheimer's Association.
Tylenol® is a registered trademark of McNeil Consumer & Specialty Pharmaceuticals

Published by North Star Books
P.O. Box 589
Pearblossom, California 93553-0589 U.S.A.
E-mail: NorthStarBooks@avradionet.com

Library of Congress Cataloging-in-Publication Data
Avadian, Brenda.
"Where's my shoes?" : my father's walk through Alzheimer's / Brenda Avadian.
    p. cm.
Summary: "A real-time telling of caregiving experiences for families worldwide who deal with Alzheimer's dementia. Topics include: Diagnosis, Support Groups, Conservatorship, In-Home & Medical Care, Skilled Nursing Care, Family Conflicts, and Legal & Financial Issues"--Provided by publisher.
  Includes bibliographical references and index.
  ISBN-13: 978-0-9632752-4-0 (pbk.)
  1. Avadian, Martin, 1910-2001--Mental health. 2. Alzheimer's disease--Patients--Biography. 3. Alzheimer's disease--Patients--Family relationships.
I. Title.
  RC523.2.A93 2005
  362.196'831'0092--dc22
                    2005006967

First edition hardback published in 1999.

9 8 7 6 5 4 3 2 1

Printed in the United States of America
Photo Credits and Captions:
Front cover photographer: Brenda Avadian. Model: Lew Jurey.

To my father, Martin Avadian,
who taught me the value of perseverance.

And to all caregivers and those who walk with Alzheimer's.

CONTENTS

PREFACE

This is the story of my father's walk through Alzheimer's. In 1996, I joined him on what would be a five-year journey. Together we learned to communicate and love unconditionally, to cope with our circumstances, and to be more patient and compassionate. Through it all, my honesty and integrity were tested repeatedly. Our lives were forever altered.

As the days added up to weeks and the weeks grew into months, my carefully constructed corporate communication and leadership-consulting career metamorphosed into that of *family caregiver*. I was lost. Even common sense evaded me. The only caregiving experience I had was taking care of cats.

While trying to meet the daily challenges of caring for my father, I was fortunate to be among a support group of caregivers. *They were walking on the same road as me!* We formed deep and meaningful relationships. We helped one another at each step of our loved ones' journeys and shared what we learned from our own experiences and from community-based and Internet resources.

"Where's my shoes?" is the (grammatically incorrect) question my father asked repeatedly as he struggled to live with Alzheimer's. I wrote this book to help those thrust into the turmoil of caring for a loved one, as I was. I want to help you be aware of your options so you can make informed decisions. Through the detailed pages that follow, I hope my father's and my experience will alleviate your feelings of loneliness, which can be overwhelming as you care for your loved one.

As Alzheimer's took away my father piece by piece, I struggled to hold on and to understand this debilitating disease. With the essence of who he was growing ever transparent and slipping away, I kept a private journal each day to make sense of what was happening to both of us.

"Where's my shoes?" is the unique telling of the caregiving journey as it occurs. Instead of recalling details years later with the benefit of hindsight, each chapter unfolds in the present moment. In this way, it preserves the poignancy and freshness of each experience *as it happens*—the same way you are walking your own caregiving journey. By sharing my experience, we can walk together as you care for your loved one.

Since the release of the first edition of *"Where's my shoes?"* in 1999, the book has sold internationally and has been translated into several languages. It is also available as an audiobook.

During this time, research has been closing the gap on the causes of Alzheimer's. This is monumental when you consider that up until the late 1990s, diagnoses were highly uncertain and families had little information with which to prepare for long-term care. For an estimated eighteen million people worldwide, each day brings more hope. Earlier diagnosis will give families the option of taking steps to delay the progression of Alzheimer's. For every month a loved one can independently carry on activities of daily living, financial costs to families and communities are reduced significantly. More importantly, the human cost of caregiving is diminished noticeably.

Readers and listeners around the world have asked about my father, my siblings, and the legal obstacles we crossed. This completely revised and expanded second edition completes my father's walk through Alzheimer's, and includes never-before-released excerpts from my father's journals, conversations with my siblings, and answers to many questions.

In honor of my father, Martin Avadian, and the eighteen million people worldwide who bravely walk this journey, the sales proceeds from this and my other Alzheimer's-related books, will help people with Alzheimer's and their families.

ACKNOWLEDGMENTS

As with any worthy endeavor, the contributions of others helped make this book a success. The following groups and people contributed to this second edition:

Antelope Valley Authors Network, whose members' experiences continue to inspire me.

Antelope Valley Care Center and its caregivers, who still welcome me and give me one more way to remember my father.

Evelyn Daniel, for some "old school" grammar tips for this edition.

Kevin Fisher, for our Website: www.TheCaregiversVoice.com

Lew Jurey, cover photo model.

Kaiser Permanente Antelope Valley Bereavement Group, who helped me express my father's enduring legacy.

Melanie Rigney, whose comments as editor at *Writer's Digest*, inspired this much-improved second edition.

Julia Ryan, whose heart-captivating cover design symbolizes the completion of my father's journey.

Support Group members at the Lancaster Adult Day Health Care, my second family, who continue to walk this road with their loved ones.

Mary Jo Zazueta, whose editing helps me become a better writer and whose page design enhances the words on each page.

Finally, David Borden, my husband and partner of twenty-seven years, who joined me on this caregiving journey and whose support enables stories about my father's walk through Alzheimer's to reach caregivers around the world.

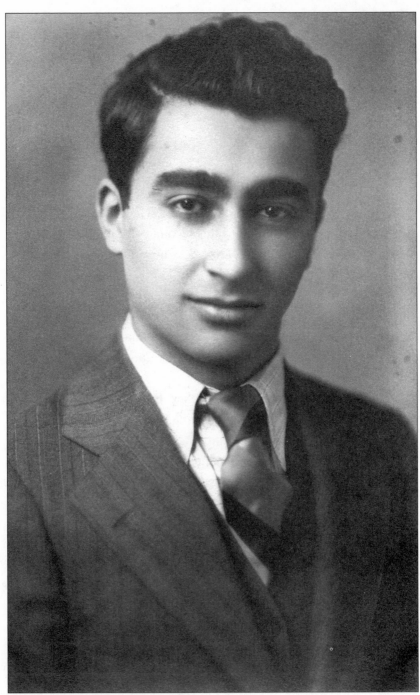

Martin Avadian at eighteen. Chicago.

ONE

In the Beginning

Martin Avadian lived through the most dynamic period in history. He lived through two world wars, the Korean War, Vietnam, and Desert Storm; and he welcomed in the new millennium. Although fiercely patriotic, he was too young to serve in World War I and was not called to serve in World War II. He witnessed massive technological changes during his ninety years on earth, from the Spirit of St. Louis to Neil Armstrong walking on the moon; from handwritten letters mailed with two-cent stamps to virtually free electronic mail arriving across the world in seconds!

Born in 1910 in Van, a prosperous predominately Armenian city in the Ottoman Empire, Martin was eight years old when his father was declared missing-in-action during the Armenian genocide. Two years later, he and his mother sailed to the United States, where they processed through Ellis Island and settled in Chicago with his mother's sister. His mother soon remarried and had two more sons.

Martin was a diligent student with an insatiable appetite for learning. He wanted to continue his schooling, but money was scarce and he didn't want to take advantage of his stepfather. So he began his independence by working odd jobs, doing anything a young teenager could do to earn money.

Martin was a private man and a hard worker. After years of working jobs for meager wages, he was hired as a machinist at General Electric. He saved money at a feverish rate. His investment strategy was conservative and consistent. During the 1950s, earning $100-plus a week, he withdrew $10 from every paycheck to buy U.S. Savings Bonds. He also accumulated General Electric stock over the years. During the 1990's stock market boom, his shares appreciated over $100,000 in less than a year. His attorneys and accountant asked, "How could a machinist accumulate so much?"

A long-time bachelor, he married at the age of thirty-nine, started a family, and moved to Milwaukee, Wisconsin. He paid cash (plus a $3,000 loan from his mother that he paid back in two weeks) for the finest home on the block owned by a banker.

While growing up, I used to gaze at his high school graduation picture that sat untouched in a gray wooden frame on the majestic oak mantelpiece of our home. I tried to imagine what kind of person he was nearly fifty years before I was born. Looking through his files, I found pictures of a gentleman, five-feet, six inches tall and 145 pounds, who prided himself on his stylish clothing and immaculate grooming. The years that followed, spanning almost a half-century, would take away much of his hearing and shrink his body to a meager five-feet-one-inch at only 112 pounds.

CHAPTER 1

The Telephone Call

"**B**renda, how are you? I hope I'm not interrupting anything. I'm calling to let you know Ma died."

WHAT? Is this real? I quickly weigh a couple thoughts. First, my father never calls me—too expensive to talk long distance—so I phone him every month. Second, is he kidding me? This is April Fools' Day—a day when people play practical jokes on each other. I decide not to be a victim of his joke.

"You've got to be kidding!" I exclaim.

"No," comes his somber reply.

"C'mon, it's April Fools' Day. Whad' ya tryin' to pull?"

"I couldn't believe it myself when the nurse called only one hour after I left her," he says with an awkward chuckle.

My mother had an enlarged heart. It was so weak it could not pump enough blood to prevent her lungs from filling with fluids. My brother, who lived with my parents, and my sister, who lived five blocks away, were frequently called to rush Ma to the hospital.

Struggling to fill her lungs with air, our mother nearly died eleven times. Swerving between lanes of cars, my brother or sister would speed through stop signals, trying to arrive at the hospital before Ma gasped her final breath. Our mother hated the noise and commotion of ambulances and refused to ride in them, saying she'd rather die instead. So, my sister and brother became her private ambulance service. After the doctors drained the fluid from Ma's lungs and increased the doses of several of the seven different medications she took three or four times a day, our mother managed to get around, albeit slowly.

I never served on this emergency transportation team, since I moved to California in 1989. From 1,800 miles away, I could only imagine these incredibly scary times with the help of my sister's vivid and sometimes teary-eyed descriptions. Ma usually insisted that my sister take her, because my brother worked farther away from home. However, my sister's inability to handle this kind of stress made us wonder if she would be admitted to the emergency room next.

Because our father was older and less able to hear and pay attention, my older sister and brother felt guilty if they didn't take Ma shopping and to her doctor's appointments.

Whenever my husband and I visited my parents, we'd also drive Ma to her appointments. These were memorable experiences for me, because Ma was a highly opinionated passenger. Oftentimes she'd lean forward, holding onto the dash, while criticizing my driving. *"Skoosh! Aman, che des-ar aht autohn? Seerd-us! Beedie merr-neem!"* she'd complain in Armenian. ("Be careful! Oh my, didn't you see that car? My heart! I'm going to die!") Even though these complaints added stress while driving, I liked helping her. Maybe I was a glutton for punishment.

Ma had a strong influence over us. Her petite and frail appearance defied her stalwart will. She was a hard worker, a *khordzavor*, as she'd say in Armenian. Others described her as resembling Mother Teresa. Her small stature, wrinkled face, rough hands, slightly stooped humbled stance, and sweet and gentle demeanor, especially with strangers, was so endearing, she could get away with almost anything.

Throughout our upbringing, I watched her befriend the most diverse populations of living beings—including schoolteachers, tattooed bikers, hippies, and doctors. Even wild animals would become docile around her.

After David and I moved to California, I kept track of my mother's progress by calling her at home and at the hospital. When Ma was in intensive care, the nurses would hold the phone to her ear while we talked. So, I was quite surprised once when I called the Intensive Care Unit and the nurse said Ma checked out nearly two weeks ago! I asked if she was transferred to another area of the hospital. "No, the doctor said there was nothing more they could do for her." I immediately thought Ma died and no one had told me. But then I remembered the pact my sister and I had made: *No matter what comes between us, we agree to give each other major news.* For some reason, she did not tell me that Ma was placed in a skilled nursing facility.

For ten years, I struggled with the uncertainty of whether our mother would survive another episode. Each time, a little piece of my heart would tear as I imagined life without Ma. After all, she raised my sister, brother, and me while my father worked two jobs outside the home. She greeted us each day after school. And, once we were grown, Ma kept the family together by keeping in touch with each of us. But lately I could sense that her personality was changing under the influence of all the medications. Formerly very active, concerned, and caring, she was bed-ridden and depressed. She spent her days complaining about all the things she could no longer do.

Still on the phone, my father continues, "In fact, I thought the nurse was kidding me and I told her so! But she assured me that when she came back into Ma's room Ma had passed away."

"Wow." *Do I feel like a fool!* "Mardig, how are you doing?" (We called my father by his first name, Martin. In Armenian, it is pronounced MAR-deeg, with the emphasis on the first syllable.)

I try focusing on my father and his feelings in an effort to postpone the jumble of thoughts in my mind and the sickening feeling in my heart. After valiantly fighting for her life for over a decade, our mother dies in Milwaukee on April 1, 1993—April Fools' Day.

"Well, under the circumstances, I'm doing all right. I'm just a bit surprised."

My father, the diplomat, the gentleman, and master of controlling his emotions. "Well, I'll fly back to visit you then. What do you need?"

"Oh, no. Don't come. You're working. Don't take time off from work."

My father worked at General Electric for thirty-two years without a single day of absence. He received special recognition for this rare achievement.

"Mardig, I will come. This is not a decision for you to make. I will help you with Ma. Besides, our family must be together during this time."

"No, that's not necessary. I have taken care of everything."

"Oh yeah? What have you done?"

We go back and forth, playfully quarreling, until he finally agrees to let me return to help him and to spend time with him.

Mardig had not made all the arrangements. In fact, he asked me to accompany him to the funeral home and cemetery. "Since you're already here, you might as well be put to work," he teased. David, who was already in Northern Wisconsin, soon joined me.

I wanted to make this a family event, so I called my sister and brother, inviting their involvement. When I reached them directly, they were "too busy" and suggested I handle the details. When I left messages, they didn't return my calls.

So, Mardig, David, and I set out to do the best we could to honor my mother's wish to be cremated. Although Mardig had already purchased a niche for both of them; he wanted Ma's ashes at home for a while.

The three of us talked about holding a family gathering. We

considered scattering some of Ma's ashes under the two evergreen trees she planted and tenderly cared for. Mardig thought this was a good idea. I called my sister and brother again, to no avail. Surprisingly, during the entire time David and I were in Wisconsin, we didn't see them. *Why did they choose to stay away?* Without them, we lost enthusiasm for a gathering. My father was disappointed, but he did not dwell upon it. I was shocked, especially at my brother, who repeatedly expressed concern about Ma's health and the quality of her care. My disappointment was long-lived. Eight years later, I would make the right decision and begin to heal.

Despite my sister and brother's failure to join our father during our time of grief, David and I moved ahead. We spent much of our time with Mardig, listening to him tell stories about his life and the places he'd like to visit. While my mother was alive Mardig felt he had to stay at home, but now we discussed a multi-country trip in October. We planned to visit Armenia—the homeland of our forebears; Moscow—a city we were curious to see; and Germany, a country my father wanted to visit having studied the language in school and where David and I could enjoy great beer during Oktoberfest.

As the time drew nearer for us to depart upon this Eastern European adventure, we feared Mardig would not go. There was nothing wrong with him. In fact, he was healthier and in better shape than I was at forty-nine years his junior! No, it was only excuses.

"Oh, I have so much to do. I have Ma's bills to pay. They're still coming, you know. I have to straighten out the house. There are papers everywhere, needing to be organized. I still have to pay taxes. The basement is a mess. I have tools laid out all over the floor. I'm afraid to go down there; it's such a big job. Once the house is straightened and I've gotten things fixed, then we'll go. What's the hurry? I'm going to live a long time!" *He was to be eighty-three that year.*

We knew better. We knew he wouldn't finish all these things. If they overwhelmed him up to this point, what would change? Instead, while we were in Milwaukee, we chartered a private plane.

Mardig had never flown, yet he was open to new experiences. We thought he'd enjoy flying. David's brother, John, a pilot at the time, flew us over Mardig's house and other recognizable landmarks—the horticultural gardens (Milwaukeeans refer to these glass dome-shaped structures as *The Three Domes*); Brewer's Baseball Stadium; and the landmark Catholic church, St. Josephat Basilica. My father enjoyed the flight and returned feeling special because we "went through all this trouble" for him.

It was only April and we knew if we remained optimistic and continued to gently persuade Mardig, he might agree to go on the Eastern European trip. Instead, his excuses flowed more frequently, up until a month before we were to depart.

I began to think about how we live conditional lives. We establish conditions upon our relationships with others and ourselves. "*If* you do this, *then* I will . . ." We also set conditions for doing things *for* ourselves, such as dining at a fine restaurant, traveling to a special place, spending time doing what we truly want to do, etc. "*If* I make a million dollars, *then* I will make time for . . ."

None of us has a guaranteed future. If we need to do something, we need to do it *now*. Other things can wait—the tools in the basement, the house being fixed, the piles of paper, and yes, even taxes! *We ended up taking care of Mardig's 1993 taxes in 1997!*

Our international adventure never got off the ground. David and I changed our approach; we invited Mardig to visit us in California. He could stay with us. He and I could spend time together after sixteen years of being apart.

For three years, we tried to persuade him to visit. When we phoned to see how he was doing, we'd have him visualize the fun he'd have in California. I drive a Mazda Miata convertible and described how he and I could go cruising the California highways with the top down. Once, when my sister and I were talking on the telephone, I mentioned how I wished I could buy Mardig new clothes. His clothes were at least twenty years old, and many were forty years old! We agreed I could *buy* him new clothes, but we knew he wouldn't *wear* them! We giggled with our visions of how he would look in a pair of khaki pants and a crisp cotton print shirt.

After my mother's passing, Mardig's life changed noticeably. David and I called every month and talked for forty-five minutes to an hour-and-a-half. These phone calls were exhausting because Mardig couldn't hear well and we had to articulate each word and speak loudly. At the end of nearly every call, I suffered from a severe headache. I wrote to him regularly so he'd have something he could read again and again for comfort. I'd include Lockheed's company newspaper when there was an article about me in it. (My father was happy when his children succeeded at work.) I sent Mardig cards for his birthday and each of the major holidays. Each year David and I flew back to Wisconsin to visit him. After a few years, we began to notice that Mardig was not taking care of himself. He was ignoring his cleanliness and nutrition. *I wondered what my brother, who still lived with him, thought of our father's worsening condition.*

Throughout his life, Mardig never cared for fancy food. If someone served it, he would eat it; but he never went to a lot of trouble preparing meals. He preferred easy-to-make foods. If you cooked him a gourmet delight, you would be disappointed with his lack of enthusiasm. A hot dog on a bun or a bologna sandwich was just fine. After Ma died, he'd walk to the neighborhood store to buy some bread and a package of bologna or hotdogs and have enough food for a week!

In contrast, Mardig always cared about his grooming; at least he did during his working years. Thanks to my mother, his clothes were always clean and neatly pressed. He showered daily, sometimes twice! He managed a very close shave and with his superb attention to detail, no stubble appeared, even in the hard-to-reach spots like his Adam's apple. He brushed his teeth for what seemed to me a long time—much longer than the dental hygienist's recommendation of two minutes. However, all this changed after our mother died. He stopped shaving and showering on a daily basis and his clothes were dirty.

Mardig was growing increasingly disoriented. From late 1994 to early 1996, David was on assignment in Wisconsin. Between his work and free time while living with his brother and sister-in-law, David juggled caring for my father. He sent me the following e-mail on a Monday in October 1995.

Dear Brenda,

I am at work and I am thinking about your father. I really think that he will soon be near the point where he will no longer be able to take care of himself. I don't think your sister or brother realizes this. Mardig doesn't talk much to them, and they really don't deal much with his day-to-day existence.

The more I think about it, I am sure your father lost about $600 this week, or it could have easily been stolen without him realizing it. It worries me somewhat that with winter coming, he may start a fire in the basement using the incinerator. He is already stockpiling wood in the basement. I really don't know why.

He really needs someone to spend time with him more and more. I know if something terrible happens to him because of his own actions, your brother and sister will wonder how he could have done something so stupid. I guess they don't really talk to him long enough or have the patience to just listen to him speak. If they'd just let him think aloud without leading the conversation, they would see that he is impaired.

I don't know what to do about this situation. I feel that I am in the middle. If I do something to try to help your father, your sister and brother will view it in a negative light because they truly see nothing wrong with him. They don't have the patience or the time to have a normal conversation with him. It is not just his hearing; it's his brain too.

I really feel he needs looking after, and I can only do so much. I was thinking of him all Saturday, Sunday, and today. It is a lot more serious than your brother and sister realize. He may end up killing himself or someone else. He really shouldn't drive anymore.

Sometimes he gets really confused and, one day, he may forget where he lives.

Sorry about this, I just needed to vent.

Love, David

Mardig began hallucinating in the months following David's e-mail. He saw my mother. He talked about my brother bringing a companion into the house. Mardig didn't know this person's name, only that he looked like my brother and he helped him carry things out of the house and spent the night when my brother was away on business. He hallucinated so vividly, we wondered if some of his visions were real.

During one of our visits, Mardig told David and me that a little girl and her friends were in the sunroom where we were sitting. "Where are they now?" I asked.

"I don't know," he said with a sheepish chuckle. "I guess they went to another part of the house when they heard the doorbell ring." *The little girl really existed. She lived with her mother across the alley behind my father's house.* Mardig shared the details with such clarity, David and I walked through the entire house before we were convinced no one else was home.

Over the following months, Mardig stopped doing things most of us take for granted. Mardig, who so meticulously attended to his grooming and appearance, completely stopped taking showers and washing his clothes.

Meanwhile, David accessed the Internet to learn what he could about Mardig's behavior. I tried getting information as well. We had difficulty understanding the information. We didn't have enough knowledge to put it all into context, nor did we know enough to know what questions to ask.

When I flew back in March of 1996, after David completed his assignment and was ready to return to California, we visited my father. We knocked on the door. Because Mardig couldn't hear well, David walked around the house to knock on the sunroom and basement windows, the two places where Mardig spent most of his time. I was surprised when the door opened quickly. I called David. My father greeted me with a big smile and welcomed me into the foyer. He asked if I was in the neighborhood. *I suppose I was, in a manner of speaking. I took a flight from Los Angeles, and after David picked me up at the airport, we came to the neighborhood to visit him.* "Yes!" I said to humor him.

"Oh, great. C'mon in! Oh, *he's* here!" Mardig added, nodding toward David, who appeared behind me. I looked at my father. He was wearing an old striped shirt soiled with dried paint and dirt. As I moved closer, I could smell him. David and I sat and talked with Mardig awhile and offered to take him to dinner. He smiled and said, "Sure, anywhere you want to go is fine with me!"

I suggested he take a shower and change his clothes first. He refused, "It's cold out. I don't want to take a shower and freeze!"

I laughed, thinking he was joking and said, "Well, you're not going to take a shower outside! You'll be inside. You'll take your shower upstairs!" He hesitated a moment and then refused with a nervous chuckle. We went out to dinner anyway. *Amazing, he no longer notices his odor or cares about wearing dirty clothes in public. My mind drifted back to my adolescence and the distinctive and unpleasant body odors of distant elderly relatives who would hug me tightly. I wondered if I would also grow old and smell.*

When we returned home, I offered to wash his clothes. "Why, when I'm working around the house and going to get dirty?" This was his humorous way of replying when he felt awkward about something. *He would not shower or let us wash his clothes during this March visit.*

The following day Mardig accepted our invitation to visit Nana, David's grandmother. He selected a short plaid wool coat to wear over his smelly clothes. Fortunately, it would mask some of the odor while hiding the dirty spots.

Nana lost her husband in 1988. When her health declined, she moved into a well-appointed assisted-living community. Maybe Mardig would consider moving into a nice place if he knew someone there. The last time we brought him, he enjoyed Nana's company, even though he forgot her a day or two later.

They were the same age. She dressed in the latest fashions, had her hair done regularly, and wore makeup highlighted with bright red lipstick. She loved to talk and my father would either sit next to or across from her and listen. He enjoyed the sight of a woman who took care of herself. Nana delighted in his company because he focused on her and smiled when she spoke. Actually, David and I agreed they made a fine couple. Mardig enjoyed looking at Nana and she enjoyed his attention. She loved to talk, and he could not hear.

We hoped Mardig would consider moving there. We knew we could never replace the void of my mother or David's grandfather who had also passed away. But, at least being of the same generation, he and Nana could keep each other company and spend their last years together, sharing lunches, social events, and dinners, while having their daily needs taken care of by the assisted-living staff.

Toward the end of our visit with Nana, we asked Mardig if he would consider living there. He was eighty-five years old. As he surveyed the dining hall and lobby, he said, "Yeah, sure would be a nice place to live once I retire!"

Chapter 2

Choices

Because Wisconsin winters are so harsh, summer is the only time of year I enjoy visiting Milwaukee. I was curious to see how Mardig lived on day-to-day basis, so I phoned him in May 1996. "Can I visit you for two weeks in July? We can celebrate the July 4th holiday together!" Although Mardig did not travel or leave the house much, I tried not to take his availability for granted.

"Noooo, why would you want to come out here?"

"We can see the fireworks together! Remember? On July third, they have the most spectacular fireworks. We can even drive on the Hoan Bridge and watch as the fireworks light up the sky over Lake Michigan!"

"Why would you waste your time with me? Don't they have fireworks where you live?" *I wasn't sure he remembered that I lived in California.*

"Yeah, they do have fireworks here, but not as spectacular as those by the lake!" I half lied.

"Naaaahhhhh, you don't want to waste your time with an old man. Don't waste your time. Go to work so you can be successful. You'll make me proud."

"Yeah, but you're my father!"

"And I'm telling you to stay home and work!" he emphasized.

Wow, he was quick with a rebuttal!

Several weeks later, when my consulting contract was extended into July, I felt relief due to Mardig's encouragement to focus on my work.

When I made my monthly call in June, I playfully asked, "Mardig, whad'ya say about my coming out to visit you in August? We can celebrate our birthdays together." *We were both born on August 22.*

Again, Mardig discouraged me. "Why are you so worried about me?"

"You're my father!"

"I am?"

This took me by surprise. "Yeah," I said hesitatingly. "You are my father and I am your daughter. Remember? Brenda?"

"Oh! Yeeaaaah!" he exclaimed.

I wasn't sure if he was joking. His question lingered in my mind as a childhood memory surfaced. My brother frequently teased me about being adopted because I was more mischievous at home and at school than he and my sister. They obeyed my parents. With a solid set of values, I was still a rebel and a handful for my parents. If I didn't look so much like my sister, I might have believed him!

"What were we talking about?" my father's question returned my attention to our phone call.

"I wanted to know if I could visit you this August."

"Why would you want to visit me?"

"So we can celebrate our birthdays together."

"Don't you have school?"

"No, I'm finished with school."

"Oh, congratulations!"

"Now, can I visit you?"

"Are you working?"

"Yea-uhh . . . yes!"

"Well, focus on your work then, so you can get ahead. You don't have to worry about me. I can take care of myself. I don't want to be a bother to you."

I paused, trying to think of a better approach. This encouragement to focus on our work was one of the underpinnings of my upbringing. Our parents came to America seeking better opportunities. As my father always said, they wanted us to "get ahead." They wanted us to live the American Dream.

My father shared his philosophy; something he did when he knew someone would listen. "Brenda, you need to understand, no one feels so important to himself that he feels he could change the course of another's life." He paused, waiting for me to digest this nugget of wisdom. It was strange, I understood him! He didn't believe I should alter my life because of him. All I wanted to do was *visit* him! I persisted. He finally gave in, "If you really want to come, you're welcome to. I just think you're wasting your time when you could be working."

One early morning, later that month, a Clinical Social Worker with the Milwaukee County Department of Aging phoned. "Are you Brenda Avadian?"

"Yes."

"Do you know a Martin Avadian?"

Concerned about the way she asked, "*a Martin Avadian*," I hesitantly replied, "Yea-uhh?" Worried that something had happened to him, I quickly added, "He's my father. Is he all right?"

"Yes, he is," she assured me. "I am calling you because something must be done for your father."

"Who are you?" I asked, since I had not paid attention when she introduced herself at the beginning of the conversation.

She repeated her name and the organization she represented.

"And you're calling me because . . . ?"

"Because something must be done for your father."

"What do you mean?" I asked, fearing they were going to take some action on him.

"Well, he could be a danger to himself."

Feeling uncomfortable, I tried to humor her, "What did he do *now*?"

She paused a moment, and without acknowledgment of my humor, explained, "Well, after visiting and evaluating him, we believe he needs assistance. Mr. Avadian called our health worker with a request to visit him. When she arrived, he asked her why she was there."

"What do you mean? You've visited him?"

"Yes, we were asked to visit him to make sure he was all right."

My mind was a blur. What a surprise! Each month I called, there was no hint others were involved. I even started journaling my father's and my monthly phone conversations shortly before I visited him in March because sometimes he'd forget or say things that didn't make sense. I didn't think it was this serious.

She continued. "He was not eating, so we arranged to have him placed on the home delivered meals program. But they can't make deliveries when he's not home. We call, and the phone rings and rings, with no answer. We come to the house and knock on the windows, we shout his name, and no one comes to the door."

"Uhh . . . did you try contacting my brother? He *lives* with *our* father!" I said with emphasis. I was surprised their interventions had gone so far and I knew nothing of them. My mind was racing. *Mardig's phone has an answering machine. Why wasn't it working? Where was my brother during all their visits? Did he have any idea?*

"Yes, I've phoned your brother many times and left messages for him at his office."

"And . . . ?"

"He has not returned my calls."

"What about my sister, then? She only lives five blocks away."

"I've also phoned her and left messages. She has not called either."

"Well, then, how did you learn about me?" I was curious since she had been working with my father awhile.

"I found your business card under the glass on his desk."

WOW! She had been in the inner sanctum—the area in the sunroom where my father does all his paperwork. This really must be serious! A sense of urgency overcame me, "Well, what can I do? You know I'm out here in California."

"We suggest you talk with your sister and brother and decide what can be done for your father."

"HAH!" I exclaimed. "Each time I come out there to visit my father, my sister says we'll get together. And then once I'm there, she says she's too busy or she doesn't return my calls."

"Well, something must be done. He may hurt himself or others. We're considering having the police do a welfare check on him, to make sure his living situation is safe. He might even have to be taken in for a psychiatric evaluation to determine his ability to live alone. *What she was saying was scary!*

"I'll come out then." *I didn't want the police involved in my father's affairs.* "I don't know what to do! Can I meet with you? Will you be able to help me?" *I feared if the state got more involved without one of us trying to help, my father would be committed to an institution. And then I could do nothing for him.*

She agreed to meet with me.

During the weeks leading to my visit, I paid closer attention to how Mardig expressed his ideas on the phone. To a stranger, he might not make sense and his comments could raise questions. When I asked him, "How are you doing?" he replied, "I'm a bit under stress. The gas and electric people are bothering me." I offered to call the utilities for him. Perhaps I could learn about the situation and try to resolve it, but he insisted on not being a problem for me. "They're going to shut off the water," he added.

"Why?" I asked.

"I made out a check for the water bill and . . . " He said he gave the check to my brother, but couldn't depend upon him. I assumed he hadn't paid the bill, and they threatened to turn off the water.

Mardig was disoriented about time. The past, present, and future seemed to coexist. His mother was living and he was a child living with her. I was a preschool child for whom he was concerned. He would cover a span of forty years in one minute!

Toward the end of one phone call, I jokingly interjected, "Where's Brenda?"

"I don't know where she is. What happened to her?"

I couldn't believe it! "I'm Brenda," I exclaimed.

"You're Brenda! You're supposed to be small! Who's your father?"

"*You* are!" I shouted, as he seemed completely involved in his world.

"Your *foster* father? Who's feeding you?" he continued. "How did he feel when you're thinking about another person—your father, whom you don't see?"

To better understand what was going on with Mardig, I frequently talked long-distance with the social worker, healthcare represent-ative, and others. I knew I had to do something, and I had many ques-tions. The difficulty was, I didn't know what questions to ask!

"How do I respond when Mardig hallucinates?"

"Kindly explain to him what is real. Be patient. Be supportive."

"What are my options for his care?"

"It depends, and this is why it's important for your sister and brother to be involved. You may want to consider assisted living." I accepted her offer to send me an informational package.

I shared my concern about my sister and brother's lack of involve-ment. She offered to contact them again to arrange a family meeting. Maybe arranging a meeting with a professional and my effort to fly back to Milwaukee, would help my brother and sister realize the ser-iousness of our father's situation.

David and I frequently discussed at length what we could do for Mardig. We talked with David's parents. We conferred with our close friends, Sally and Ken, who were taking care of Sally's father in their own home. We talked with Lew, who was about to retire and move to Mississippi with his wife, Jo, to enjoy the thirty-acre estate they just purchased. We brainstormed ideas with Dave, who earned worldwide recognition for being the first person to fly the prototype of the F-22 Raptor fighter plane, and his wife, Jan, a native Wisconsinite. These people knew us best. I was about to return to Wisconsin. A decision had to be made. *What were we going to do for Mardig?*

The week before I flew to Milwaukee, I called the social worker and learned she was unsuccessful in getting my sister and brother involved. Despite this, she and I set an appointment.

Meanwhile, I continued brainstorming all the things I needed to do before I arrived and while I was in Milwaukee. Each item I wrote spurred another item and another and my list of things to do covered many areas. I was already overwhelmed and I had not even departed!

We seriously considered having Sally care for my father. Having compassion for the elderly and being a helpful person, she was open to the possibility. Sally was caring for her eighty-something father, Pete, during his final years. Although her and Ken's burden was made greater by all the modifications they made to their home to accommodate her father's wheelchair, Pete was able to live in a nice place with his family. We addressed the specifics—Sally quitting her job to care for my father, payment, and what-ifs. For example, what if she quit her established job with full benefits to take care of Mardig and he died in two months? What would happen to her income requirements? What if she and Ken wanted to travel? Mardig might require a lot of attention and care, preventing them from traveling.

After a number of in-depth and honest discussions, we mutually agreed this was not a reasonable option given Sally and Ken's plans.

What was I going to do? Witnessing my confusion and uncertainty, Sally loaned me a book, *How Did I Become My Parents' Parent?*, by Harriet Sarnoff Schiff. She said it helped her with her father. I devoured it voraciously. I needed all the information I could get. I would be in Milwaukee for only two weeks. I wanted to *do something* for Mardig.

After talking with distant relatives and friends, and reading information sent by the social worker and others; David and I came up with four options.

1. Arrange for a caregiver to look after Mardig a few hours each day as needed. We were hesitant about this option because we did not know much about the services provided by geriatric care managers or even the dependability of a paid caregiver.

What if the caregiver didn't show up one day? What if the caregiver abused my father? How would we monitor quality or dependability of care from 1,800 miles away? After all, my brother *lived* in our father's home and Mardig still needed assistance.

2. Move Mardig into an assisted-living community near his home. This would keep him in a familiar city. However, given his reaction when we visited Nana in March, we wondered if he would ever see himself as retired in order to enjoy a nice place like hers. Or, we could move him into an assisted-living community in California. Years ago, my mother and father took cross-country trips to California because they dreamed of living in a warmer climate. Perhaps we could help my father live his dream.

3. Mardig could live with us. David and I have no children. We lead active lives and are intensely involved with our professions, which requires us to travel. We eat one meal a day between rushing from one activity to the next. Anytime we discussed starting a family, we faced an obstacle. Our old-fashioned values included one of us staying home to raise our children. We didn't want to bring children into the world only to have someone else raise them. In the nineteen years we'd been together, the only children in our lives were of the independent feline variety.

4. Do nothing. During our monthly phone conversations and annual visits, my father frequently reminded us of his independence. He repeatedly turned down our offers to assist him, and was surprised we thought he needed help. He believed he was doing fine. Yet, Milwaukee winters produce freezing, razor-sharp winds that lash deeply into exposed skin. As Mardig grew increasingly disoriented, he might get lost one day and freeze to death. We figured I would simply go back to Milwaukee, enjoy the time I spent with Mardig, create some memories, and then return home. This might even be the last time I see him alive. *Let my brother and sister worry about him. My brother LIVES WITH HIM! My sister lives five blocks away.*

Why should I be concerned when I live more than 1,800 miles away? Besides, I'm the youngest child and the first one who permanently left home! If Mardig causes serious danger to himself or others, like running an old space heater too close to his blankets and starting a fire, he'll be evaluated and then placed in a county facility. If my sister and brother refuse to help, Mardig will become a ward of the state. *What a tragedy.*

These options spun around in our minds. David and I lost sleep thinking of them. And then David reminded me of the time in 1991 when we adopted a rat.

While sitting outside on the patio, we spotted a dirty white rat. It took a few steps along the back fence, made a squeaky noise, took a few more steps, and then made another noise. We tracked it, wondering how a rat had managed to find our backyard, since we live in a tract housing area with newer homes divided by six-foot wooden fences. David tried getting the rat's attention by mimicking its squeaky noises, but it fell to the other side of the fence where a Doberman pinscher lived. David ran inside the house, opened a can of cat food, and came outside with a bowl and spoon to coax the rat to our side of the fence before it became dog food. Squeaking like the rat, David encouraged it to return, while generously spooning half the can's content into a bowl on the patio. The rat was nowhere to be found. We went inside the house to put the remaining cat food away and to get a snack when we heard sounds on the patio. We looked to find the rat standing by the bowl, sniffing the food. We paused and then slowly opened the patio door to get a closer look.

It looked at us a moment, then turned toward the food and immediately began to gorge itself. David and I watched as this rodent's sides expanded with each swallow. The poor thing must have been starved. I'd only seen white lab rats before. Sitting a couple feet away, I examined its features. This rat was larger than I first thought. It was scraggly; its pink tail was covered with strands of wiry fur; and its ears were pitted, bloody, and scabbed with black dots inside. The rat ate all the food and looked up at us, as if to assess its benefactors. Then it squeaked some more. I reached down hesitatingly to pet it and was able to feel its fur before it jittered cautiously away. Its fur felt dry and wiry. David went inside to get more cat food. As David spooned another quarter can into the bowl, the rat approached and continued to eat ravenously. As its sides expanded, I exclaimed, "David, you'd better stop feeding it. It might explode!" He laughed and agreed. He petted it before it moved a distance and watched us.

We went inside to wash the bowl and our hands before returning outside. David set out a fresh bowl of water. Sitting on the patio, I asked, "David, what are we going to do with this thing? We can't keep it!" The two stray cats we adopted in 1987 while living in Wisconsin would not tolerate this! They took over the house and hissed each time the neighbors' cats came into our yard. I hated to think what they would do with an oversized rat!

"Well, we'll feed it and see what happens."

"No, *you'll* feed it," I emphasized.

"Do you mind?" David asked.

"No," I sighed.

We are such softies when it comes to animals and even insects. They'll be given a safe place to stay, provided they don't scratch or bite us.

David set food outside each day, and the rat returned to eat. As the days passed, the rat grew fur and gained weight. Fur even covered its tail and ears. Two weeks later, we realized we had not adopted a rat, but a CAT!

We took it to the veterinarian, who said it was a six-pound, full-grown spayed female with lots of ear mites. The vet and technician both laughed when they heard our rat story.

We brought her home, and David gave her a bath. The cat was not amused. David survived. We gave her the name, Djermag, "white" in Armenian.

Reflecting on this, David and I realized if we would consider adopting a rat, we needed to reevaluate our priorities. *After all, this man is MY FATHER! We have to do something for MY FATHER!*

CHAPTER 3

My Last Visit?

In August, I opened the front screen door and knocked on the oak door. What a surprise when my father opened it immediately. Greeting me with a big smile, he said, "It's good to see you! Were you in the neighborhood?"

"Yes," I muttered, distracted by what I saw. He was wearing the *same* striped shirt he had worn five months earlier when we saw him in March. Except this time, it was dirtier and several of the buttons were unbuttoned. As he stood there, stooped from eighty-six years of life's burdens, I could see darkened skin near his collarbones. As I moved closer, pungent body odor flooded my nostrils. I realized he was dirty. It was a hot and humid 85-degree day in Milwaukee. I knew my father had not showered or changed his clothes since March. How sad. My father lived in his own home for forty-five years and he looked and smelled worse than a homeless person! *What was I to do?*

Before I departed for Milwaukee David and I weighed each of the four options. We settled on two. First, I'd see if Mardig would agree to move into an assisted-living community. If this didn't work, I'd spend memorable time with him and then return home. Finally, as his health deteriorated, the state would step in. We assumed my sister and brother had little interest in Mardig or his affairs.

In spite of not returning our calls, and not supporting or offering to help when I did talk with them, I remained optimistic. David said I was knocking my head against a brick wall. I phoned my sister and she answered the telephone. I shared the four options we were considering. Surprisingly, she said she'd support my decision. "Would you be willing to help?" I asked.

"How so?" *This was a shock.*

"You could help convince Mardig to move into an assisted-living facility," I eagerly offered. We weighed the risks of Mardig living safely at home versus the stress of moving him out of the home he'd occupied for nearly a half-century. *Maybe if I involved her in the decision process, she'd eventually get involved.*

"I'll think about it," she said.

Encouraged, I called Mardig. I didn't expect my brother to answer the phone, but he did. Excited about the possibility of my sister helping, I told my brother about the option of placing Mardig in an assisted-living facility. Without hesitation he loudly retorted, "Mardig doesn't want to go into a nursing home!" Mardig must have been in the kitchen with him because I heard him say, "Hey, Mardig! Brenda wants to put you in a nursing home. You wanna go?" This was his style of humor. And then he added, "We're busy right now. Good-bye," and hung up the phone. Still holding the receiver, I sat dumbfounded.

Since I would leave for Milwaukee after Mardig's and my birthday, David and I celebrated at home. Then we phoned Mardig to sing a humorous, harmonious rendition of "Happy Birthday."

The following day, August 23, I was awakened by a phone call at 5:39 a.m. *We always answer the phone because we never know when an emergency call might come.*

"We have to talk!" the voice demanded, slicing into my sleep. "Are you awake?"

"Ugh . . . yeah . . . yes . . . yeah . . . I'm awake," I replied, trying to make sense of what I was hearing. I had stayed up until the pre-dawn hours, brainstorming the strategic direction of our sideline business with our partners. Thinking about the exciting prospects for getting subscribers to the only television network devoted exclusively to personal and professional development, had made it difficult for me to sleep.

"Mardig's been wandering the streets all night since one o'clock. He came here at seven a.m. I told him to go home. I don't want him here!" It was my sister. Her words chiseled into my rapidly waking mind. "Two days ago, the police picked him up."

Did something happen to Mardig? Why was she calling me so early?

She sounded angry, and I was tired. Every time something went wrong, she explained, people called *her*—the authorities, Mardig, social service workers. Every time she tried to contact my brother, he rebuffed her. "I-want-to-see-him-in-a-home!" She shouted each word distinctly.

I couldn't take it any longer. *Each time I suggested we work together, she said she was too busy. Now, she was calling me because she had a problem. Well, I was tired!* "Why are you calling me?" I asked.

Just then, I heard her husband say Mardig was at their door again. My sister shouted, "I don't want him in this house! Tell him, 'Don't come here anymore!'"

My sister was placed in a no-win situation. She asked Mardig for keys to his house so she could more easily help him in an emergency. He would not give her the keys. When he lost his keys or locked himself out, he went to her. If our brother were unreachable, she'd help Mardig get into the house by breaking a window or some other means.

Reasoning that if I offered to help her with *her* problem, she might be more willing to work with me, I asked, "How can I help?"

She shouted, "I don't want anything to do with Mardig! I don't care if he dies! I am sick of taking care of his problems. I have problems of my own. I helped take care of Ma and got nothing!" *Our brother, who also helped care for our mother, managed to get a sizable sum of money transferred to his account. My sister felt shortchanged and unappreciated for her efforts.*

After the phone call ended, I sat up awake, aghast. "Why? Why does it have to be like this?"

Standing in the foyer of my father's home, I felt uncomfortable. The sun was shining outside, while the inside of the house was dark. Musty air filled my nostrils. For the first time in my life, claustrophobia closed in as the still, warm air surrounded me in the darkness.

"Are you hungry?" My father's question pulled me out of my thoughts.

"Uh-uh, nah," I stuttered.

"Well, come in then and have a seat," he motioned me toward the kitchen, ignoring my response. The kitchen curtains and shade were closed, so I turned on the light. The stagnant air made it difficult to breathe. "Why don't we sit outside?" I suggested. He agreed. I followed him out to the back of the house. He walked across the backyard to the garage. He unlocked the door and went inside.

I looked around. The house looked worn. Contrasting white mortar patched the loose brickwork in some areas, and gray sealant filled the cracks in the white cement sidewalk and steps. The grandeur of what was once a bank president's home was gone. My father was the second owner of this one-and-a-half-sized city lot that was in desperate need of attention.

The garden had long been unattended. It was now an overgrown array of wild weeds and flowers, with the exception of four trees—my father's famous apple tree, my mother's pear tree, and the two evergreen seedlings my mother planted shortly before her death. The evergreens were about a foot tall when she planted them; now they stood over eight feet high. I could only guess what flora and fauna inhabited the overgrown urban ecosystem.

My thoughts went back many years to when my mother watered her vegetable garden. I enjoyed sitting on these steps smelling the freshly watered plants. Sometimes, when the wind blew just right, a light cool mist would tickle me.

Mardig returned with two soiled foam pads. He placed them on the cement steps to the back door of the house. After looking at the paint and oil stains on the gold-colored foam pads I seriously considered sitting directly on the cement. But I accepted his kind gesture and sat down next to him. We talked about whatever came into his mind. We began with names of family members, how they were related, and who was still living. He couldn't remember, so I helped him recreate our family. He complimented me on knowing so much about our family. But even I got confused when he referred to "Ma" each time he spoke about *his* mother and *my* mother. We talked awhile, then he reminded me his lunch would be delivered before 1:00 p.m. He didn't want to miss it.

We got up and Mardig carried the cushions to the front steps of the house. I ran inside to get a few sheets of scrap paper and a clipboard. I wanted to create a family tree for him as we reviewed once more our family members' names and their relationships. I joined him at the front of the house and we talked about each family member as I wrote the name and linked each relationship on paper. He watched and showered me with more compliments. When I downplayed his praises, he insisted, "No, really, you know a lot about our family! Even I don't remember all these people!"

A small, unmarked white truck pulled up in front of the house and I quickly rose and ran down the stairs to get his meal. Introducing myself as Mardig's daughter, I thanked the delivery woman. She was happy he was home, because Mardig often missed his meals. I ran up the stairs and my father and I walked inside so he could eat.

We sat at the kitchen table. He invited me to share his meal. It was a single serving chicken entrée with a vegetable side dish, a roll, dessert, milk, and apple juice. I declined, wanting him to eat his food. He insisted. I feared if I did not at least take one bite, he would feel funny eating alone and stop. He put a forkful of vegetables in his mouth and got up to get a couple slices of bread. He loved soft white bread. "Easy on the teeth," he'd say. Neither he nor I wanted the milk or the apple juice, so I suggested we get something else to drink.

I opened the refrigerator. All I saw was a gallon of milk and a half-gallon of orange juice on the top shelf and another half-gallon container sitting on the bottom in a putrid-smelling pool of liquid drainage from the refrigerator. The orange juice on the top shelf had my brother's name printed on it. I retrieved the juice from the bottom shelf, taking care to hold a paper towel underneath it. I noticed the expired date on the container and felt sick with shame. My brother lives in our father's home, while *his* father has to depend on a county program for his daily nourishment. I drained the contents into the sink. Mardig objected loudly. Ignoring him, I crushed the empty plastic container with my foot and threw it in the trash.

Mardig could get sick from eating spoiled food. He's older and would not recover easily. I continued looking elsewhere in the kitchen. The cupboards were stuffed with plastic grocery bags and empty foil trays, the same ones used for his home-delivered meals. I bent down to look into the lower cabinets. Reaching in, I retrieved plastic bags filled with off-colored rice. I opened the kitchen curtain and raised the shade to see pink-tinted rice. *Pink rice? Is there such a thing? I've had white rice (long and short grain), glutinous, Basmati, and brown rice . . . I'd never seen pink rice before.* The plastic bags were sticky, a sign they had been there awhile and were degrading. I reasoned they had been there while my mother was alive. I took all the bags, poked a hole in them, and let the rice drain into the kitchen garbage container. My father was disgusted with me and complained, "You're wasting all this good food!"

"I want to go grocery shopping because there's nothing to eat in this house!" I retorted.

"Yeah, because you're throwing it all away!" he shouted cynically.

"Besides, I *need* a beer!"

"A beer? That's no good for you."

In my lifetime, I never saw my father taste alcohol. In fact, until my sixth grade teacher brought us a bottle of cognac after visiting Russia, there wasn't any alcohol in our home. *I wonder if it's still there.* I stood on a chair to look in the cabinet above the refrigerator where my parents stored the cognac. I remember wanting to sneak a taste once, but it was sealed. I'd get into trouble if the seal were broken. I remained curious and every time I had a sore throat, I'd tell my mother that other kids' parents used a spoonful to heal their sore throats. During a weak moment, she let me try it. One spoonful was all I got. YUCK! It tasted worse than the cough medicine!

My sixth grade teacher was one of my two favorite elementary schoolteachers. Except for a little tremor, her penmanship was perfect, like the green penmanship cards with white letters stuck above chalkboards in schools. She was surprised to discover my handwriting was better than hers. When I got into trouble and my mother banished me to my bedroom, I'd practice my penmanship. I'd come downstairs early to seek her approval; and because she valued neat writing, she did not force me to go back upstairs.

After my teacher broke her writing arm, she asked me to write for her. I stood at the front of the class and wrote on the chalkboard when she asked. She even asked me to stay after school a couple times to help her write checks. At eleven years of age, I'd never seen a check before. My parents only used cash. I felt so special because, unlike all the other times, this time I had to stay after school because my help was genuinely needed. After the first time, I ran home to tell my mother. She was proud of me and she geared up to help my teacher. She offered to go to her house and help her. My mother was doing good things for my teachers. Her deeds never seemed to impact my conduct grades, however. I still got into trouble for talking too much, giggling, or getting into other kinds of harmless but disruptive mischief.

"Hey, what are ya lookin' for?" my father asked.

"Oh, nothing, it's not there."

"Well, I didn't take anything. Everything's been the way Ma left it."

Yes, I know! The rice, the bags, and who knows what else!

"Mardig, I need to go food shopping."

"I'll come with you. You're my guest and I want you to be comfortable."

He quickly finished his meal and took another sip of his water. I drank the rest of my water and finished the half slice of bread I'd taken. I reminded him, "We need to go to the store."

"Okay, wait a minute," he said, getting up and walking away, leaving the foil tray and breadcrumbs scattered on the table. "I have to get my wallet, because we'll need money."

"You don't need money, Mardig," I said, calling after him. "We're just going to pick up a few things. Besides I'm going to get some beer."

Returning, he said, "You don't need any beer, but you're my guest, I'll pay." Then he left the room.

I waited nearly ten minutes as I tossed the foil container in the trash, wiped the tabletop, closed the loaf of bread, and washed our cups and utensils. He returned, apologizing. He had misplaced his wallet and had to look for it.

We went to the store. As we walked up and down each aisle, I asked, "Mardig, what do you want?" Or, I'd point to something, "Do you want this?"

"Whatever you want, I'll eat anything as long as you make it."

We quickly made the rounds and picked up a variety of easy-to-prepare items.

At the checkout line, Mardig looked inside his wallet. The total came to nearly thirty dollars; he only had eleven. He insisted on giving me ten, explaining he had to save one dollar in case of an emergency. I added a twenty-dollar bill to his ten, and took the receipt. He pushed the cart of groceries outside to the car.

We had bologna, fresh bread, chocolate pudding, an assortment of chewy cookies, milk, orange juice, bananas, grapes, tomatoes, soda, and, for me, bottled beer. His refrigerator was now better stocked. Even I could nibble on a few things.

Mardig wanted to visit my sister. "I don't get to see you two together," he explained.

"Let's call her," I suggested. *If we just appeared at her door, she would not open it. She had not returned my calls, letters, or e-mails during the months prior, and even though I traveled many miles to be in Milwaukee, she was "too busy" to visit.*

"All right, call her," he said.

"No," I said. I wasn't in the mood to be rejected. "If you want to visit her, you call her. She will respond better to you."

He called her. Since he was hard of hearing, he found it easier to hear through the speakerphone. I stood quietly by his side as the answering machine played her telephone greeting (she screened her calls). When he heard her voice, he began talking. When my sister's voice continued, he became confused and flustered. After the long beep, he managed to leave a message.

We then went into the sunroom, where he started shuffling papers on his desk.

The phone rang. I asked Mardig to get it. I listened to see if it was for me, since I had given his number to the social worker and to my friends. It was my sister. If she sounded friendly and pleasant, I would talk with her.

"Mardig, are you all right?" she asked.

"Yes."

"Wha'cha doin'?" she asked playfully.

"I have company."

"Who?"

I pointed to myself and shook my head no. Mardig did not divulge my identity.

"Come here and see."

"Mardig, who?" she inquired, sounding concerned.

"Come and see!" he toyed, holding his ground.

"Mardig, I have things to do!" she replied in an irritated manner.

"C'mon, just for a few minutes," he pleaded. (She lived only five blocks away.)

"Mardig, I have to take [her husband] to work."

This went nowhere. I was glad I didn't answer the phone. I had heard these excuses too many times before. Even while I write this, my anxiety increases and I feel my muscles tighten. Excuses, excuses, excuses!

Mardig and I returned to the sunroom. As he looked over the paperwork on his desk, I asked, "Mardig, why don't you consider moving into the place where Nana lives?"

"Where?" he asked, still looking at his papers.

"You know, that place we visited in March, with David. His grand-ma lives there and you enjoy spending time with her."

"Yeah," he turned to me and smiled and then pointed at his desk, "once I finish all this work around the house. I can't just leave it, you know."

"Well, you can live there and take some of this work with you. They'll prepare your meals and even wash your clothes while you finish your work." I didn't know if this was true, but it made me feel good to consider it. I didn't even know if they would be able to accommodate his hobby working on small motors and other electrical items. But, I reasoned, if his basic needs were taken care of he could at least catch up on his paperwork.

"Nah, that would be too much trouble. Besides, my food is easy, just a bun and a hot dog is all I need."

"Well, what if someone comes and lives with you?"

Chuckling, he looked at me. "Why would someone want to do that?" Pausing, as if to ponder this, he added, "They would only get in the way!"

"Mardig, I'm concerned for you. It's getting harder for you to manage everything by yourself."

"You got that right." As he swiveled in his chair, he added, "Yeah, I'm getting behind around the house here." Pausing again, he started shaking his head. "Maybe later, once I'm finished with everything around this house."

"Mardig," I risked irritating him, especially after the earlier food-tossing episode, but he needed to be aware, "Remember you got lost and the police had to bring you home?"

"What? When?" he asked, looking right at me, genuinely surprised. Chuckling nervously, "I haven't done anything with the police!"

I pushed a little more, "Mardig, did you know a Milwaukee County social worker is helping you? She's making sure you're managing all right."

He laughed with disbelief. "Me? Why would all these people be concerned about me?"

"Well, there's no food in your refrigerator, you got lost, and they consider you a risk to yourself and possibly others. What if one day, while you're walking home from the bank, some kids who want to have a little fun, hurt you? And besides," recounting the reason my sister called one pre-dawn morning, "you might freeze to death if you lock yourself out of your house."

Chuckling and shaking his head, Mardig took a deep breath and gave me his perspective. "Millions of people die each year. We're like animals . . . we keep crawling until we stop."

Wow, his comment floored me! I couldn't believe what he just said. I was shocked. I disagreed. I gulped and then spewed forth, "Mardig, I can't accept this. You're a human being. We are different from animals. You are my FATHER!"

He looked at me with earnest eyes, "After I die it doesn't matter."

What should I do? If we moved him out of his home, he might die because he had nothing to live for. At least, in his home, things were familiar. He could tinker with his tools and work on his projects. He would have things to accomplish and feel he has a purpose. Take these away and he may lose his reason for living. Could I accept the risk of removing Mardig from the place he had called home for so long, just to be assured he would survive the winter? What if the move was too much for him to bear and he died a few months later? Would I be able to face myself then? *I wished there was someone I could call who had all the right answers.*

Fortunately, I was talking with enough people to understand this was not about me. It was not about what would be *convenient* for *me*. It had to be what was best for Mardig, what would work for him.

While in Milwaukee, I stayed with David's brother, John; his wife, Anna; and Finn, their springer spaniel. My father's home was stocked like a warehouse and lacked amenities for an overnight stay. Despite David and Anna's kindness and our occasional dinner discussions, I felt alone as my thoughts swirled at a dizzying pace. I began to feel depressed. No one *really* understood what I was going through.

The day before meeting with the social worker, I called my sister and left a message on her answering machine: "On Friday when we talked, you said you'd return my calls. I'm in Milwaukee now. The social worker has arranged a meeting for all of us at . . . Please call me at . . ." I left the phone number where she could reach me after telling her where and when the meeting would be held. I hoped she would attend this meeting. I was torn between hope and frustration. Here I was, the youngest child, living 1,800 miles away, trying to get a handle on my father's affairs. Meanwhile, my sister and brother lived *near* or *with* him and were ignoring the whole situation. I couldn't believe it!

I eagerly anticipated the meeting because I needed answers. After talking with the social and health workers and others, I prepared one-and-a-half pages of questions and issues on graph paper with enough space between each item for my notes. I was excited about having answers to each of these issues in less than twenty-four hours. I envisioned walking out of the meeting with a clear sense of direction.

I met the social worker in a large conference room with tall ceilings in an old Cream City brick building two miles from my father's house. After initial and brief pleasantries, I felt the urge to get started; I wanted to cover all of my notes. She realized she needed another file and excused herself to retrieve it. I reviewed my papers.

The first issue was a psychiatric assessment. During an earlier phone conversation, the health care worker suggested one was in order to determine my father's competence. When she returned, I asked her what it might cost. "Three hundred to three hundred and fifty dollars." *I didn't know what kind of health insurance Mardig had. I was willing to pay for the assessment, in order to get an expert's opinion as soon as possible.* She said if he was incompetent, we could go before a judge to appoint a guardian.

"Is that like a conservatorship?" I asked.

"Yes, in some states it is referred to as a guardianship and in others, a conservatorship. But there may be differences in each state. You'll have to check with an attorney to be sure."

"How would it work when my father lives in Wisconsin and I live in California?"

"Your sister and brother would have to be his guardians."

"Hah!" I blurted out, knowing this would never happen. Still, I tried to keep an open mind. "What, in your experience, would be the success in getting them to accept this role?"

"Well, they're not here. And we made repeated attempts to contact them . . . so, not good."

"What do you suggest?" I asked, looking for a quick fix.

"The state could appoint a professional to be his guardian."

"No, he would not like this. Besides, we're his family, one of us needs to be involved. What else do you suggest?"

"Looking at your family situation, you could encourage Mr. Avadian to move into an assisted-living facility."

This seemed to be the most attractive option, and I knew just the place. But how could David and I convince Mardig, especially after our previous attempts had been unsuccessful? Maybe the social worker would have a better approach.

"You could spell out the benefits for your father—twenty-four-hour staff to take care of his needs, friends with whom to socialize, activities, coordinated tours, and more."

"This sure seems like the best option, especially since my husband's grandmother lives in a nice one in South Milwaukee and my father enjoys her company. But, I do have one concern. What if my father experiences trauma after moving away from his familiar surroundings of forty-five years?"

"I agree, that is a potential risk."

"Still, he has not been paying his bills. He says the gas and electric people are after him."

"They are?" she looked concerned.

"Well-lll, yes." *I felt uncomfortable sharing private details, fearing the state might take over and then our family would have no choice in his care. My father would be disappointed that we opened his life to government oversight.*

"What do you mean?"

"I think he hasn't paid his utilities, so they're threatening to stop his service."

"Oh, I see. There is a law in the state of Wisconsin that if a disabled or ill person doesn't pay his bills . . . "

My mind trailed off in another direction and I stopped listening to her. I was getting in over my head. I looked around the conference room. It was just the two of us, my father's file in front of her and my papers in front of me, trying to determine my father's future—and he had no idea what was going on. It was strange trying to resolve my father's fate.

I looked up to see her jotting a few notes in her folder. "What about other options?" When she didn't reply fast enough, I asked, "What about having someone move in with my father to care for him?"

"That's a good idea. And you won't have to worry about him being traumatized, since he can stay in his own home." Pausing for a moment to think, she added, "Although, I wonder if your father would agree to this. He seems very independent. And then, there's your brother." Pausing again, she asked, "Does he *live* there?"

"I'm not really sure," I said, articulating each word in an attempt to get her sympathy. "Sometimes when I call my father, my brother answers the phone, so he must be home. But even when I call him at work and leave a message with his answering service, he does not return my calls. He has a business in a western suburb, and I haven't seen him at home since I've been here."

"Is this typical of families?" I asked quickly. I wanted her to express a concern for my situation and find a better way to help me. Maybe I could use her position with the county to insist my brother and sister get involved. *Or else!*

"Yes, for some this is typical, while others are different."

How depressing! I wanted to hear that our situation was unique. I wanted her to say my brother's and sister's behavior was unacceptable, and unless they got involved, the state would step in.

Since we had less than an hour, I was pressured to move to the next item on my list. I went back to the options. David and I worried about the stories we heard of live-in caregivers taking advantage of the elderly, so this would have to be a last resort.

"What other options are there? There have to be more options!"

She paused a moment. "If you're having difficulties getting your siblings involved, you could go to court and get a guardianship."

"Yeah, but they'd still need to be involved in a guardianship arrangement, otherwise the state would appoint one."

"Oh . . . right."

We had covered this before.

"What exactly is a conservatorship?"

"Well, a guardianship as we use it in Wisconsin is a court-ordered document appointing a responsible person to care for a person deemed incompetent."

This bothered me. I did not think Mardig was incompetent. At least, I wasn't ready to admit it. I wanted to preserve as much of his independence and dignity as possible. "Do you think my father is incompetent?"

"Well-uh, not really," she stammered, then quickly added, "I can't make that determination; only a doctor can."

Frustrated, I asked, "Well, just why *did* you get involved in the first place?"

"I'm not really sure what started it." She looked through her papers. "I don't have the health file here, but our office must have received reports of Mr. Avadian's disorientation, lack of proper nutrition, and possible neglect."

"Given your work with my father, where do *you* see him?"

"Mr. Avadian's on the fence, actually. He is still borderline. He can manage by himself, he just needs occasional supervision due to his dementia."

"What? What is that?"

"Dementia? It means he is losing some of his abilities."

"You mean, like his memory?"

"Yes, and he's getting increasingly disoriented."

"Yeah, I heard the police picked him up," I volunteered.

"Eventually, he won't be able to take care of himself or make decisions."

I was listening only partially. My brain was already too full and many questions remained on my list. We were only part way down the first page!

"So, he'll get worse?"

"Yes, as the disease progresses . . . " she stopped and then added, "these questions are best answered by Mr. Avadian's doctor."

"Do you know who his doctor is?"

She looked in her folder and said he had been going to the neighborhood clinic a few blocks from his home. "I don't have any more information in this folder, but you can go there and find out which doctor Mr. Avadian is seeing."

I jotted down the information and glanced quickly at my two sheets of graph paper. Surprisingly, her answers were covering the issues on the second page. Suddenly the time pressure was lifted because we were making progress. I sighed with relief and smiled. This social worker was helping me more than I thought. "What other options are there?" I asked, even though I knew I was repeating myself.

"There's the POA."

"The what?"

"Power of attorney."

"What is that?"

"Your father can appoint an attorney to act on his behalf."

"I'm not sure he has an attorney. I'm not sure he would want to pay for one."

"No," she smiled and laughed lightly. "He would give one of you power of attorney."

Is she serious? We don't have law degrees!

"Your father can appoint you to serve as his attorney for his financial affairs and health care."

"Oh, so that's what a POA is!"

In March, David and I accompanied my father to the bank because he wanted witnesses to see how much money he had. Mardig and I had been to the bank earlier in the week. He feared if he didn't check on his account, the bank would forget about him and keep his money. When we walked in, a bank representative stood immediately and greeted us from behind her desk next to the tellers' stations. Mardig had been coming to the bank almost every day, asking about his account and requesting printed copies of his balance. During our previous visit the bank representative suggested Mardig appoint me as his power of attorney. Mardig agreed to it during this subsequent visit saying he liked the way I looked out for him. It happened so fast. I signed a little card and that was the last I heard about it.

"My father granted me power of attorney over his bank account. Does this count?" I asked, giddily thinking we had already taken care of everything and I was worrying needlessly.

"No, the POAs I'm talking about are different. You'll need two of them, one for his financial and related affairs and the other for his health care."

"I'm not sure what you mean," I said, disappointed because things were never as easy as I hoped.

She explained that a power of attorney allows the appointed person to legally represent another's interests and make decisions.

My heart sank. On one hand, I felt a childlike excitement of being appointed a high level of responsibility—an "attorney" no less! After all, I was the baby of the family. The youngest family member never got any respect! Wow, I was about to do a very grown-up thing. It was like getting behind the wheel of a car for the first time. It was like buying my first house. I felt grown-up. On the other hand, I had a dreadful sinking feeling.

I felt so alone. What was I to do? I really wished my sister and brother would be involved. Since I wasn't having any luck talking directly with them, maybe there was another way the social worker could help. I shared my feelings. She said it would be better if all of us, my brother, sister, and I, encouraged Mardig to let us help him. Again, she volunteered to call my brother and sister to have them follow up with me. She suggested all of us could serve as Mardig's POA.

I liked this idea. This way, *all* of us would be involved. But the responsibilities of a shared POA require coordination and agreement. Since my brother and sister didn't return our calls, would this work?

"Is there anything else you can suggest; anything we haven't covered yet?" I was happy and felt more relaxed, her replies had answered other issues I had thought of. Hopefully, we could finish soon because my mind was reeling and I had a headache.

"First you get the POA to take care of his affairs and possibly to place him in assisted living. Then you can get a competency hearing."

"So get a POA first and then the competency hearing?"

"Yes."

"Can you recommend any attorneys?" *I had no idea where to start.*

"We can't recommend attorneys, but we do have a list of local elder law attorneys that I can give to you."

"I would like that."

"I'll have to send it to you later, because the person who has the list is not here today. In case I forget, here's her name and phone number. Call her if you don't hear from her within the next few days."

"Oh, thanks. For the competency hearing, what's involved?"

"Mr. Avadian would get a full physical and a psychological and psychiatric assessment. If he's competent, he can continue living at home, as he has been. If not, he will need a court-appointed guardian."

We discussed a few more details and then reviewed what each of us was going to do. She would contact my sister and brother *again*, talk to the lady about the list of elder law attorneys, and see if she could get more information about my father's health records. I would try to find an attorney, follow up with my father's doctor at the clinic, and see if I could get my brother and sister involved.

Ever hopeful, I called my sister. *As David would say, "Brenda, you're knocking your head against a brick wall."* She answered the phone and caught me completely off guard. I was only prepared to leave a brief message on her answering machine. "I wish you could have attended the meeting with the social worker yesterday," I said.

She showed no interest. I repeated the message I had left for her earlier about working together to determine what we could do for Mardig while I was in Milwaukee. She started listing off all the things she had to do. "Brenda, the building inspector's on my back!"

I'd heard this excuse for three-and-a-half years, even while our mother was alive! She bought older homes and fixed them up. Milwaukee either had a very patient building inspector or my sister had a very strong back!

"I'm here now. We can work together. Remember all the times you got the brunt of the requests? Remember the early morning call?"

"What phone call?"

"The one where you said Mardig was at your front door and wandering since one o'clock in the morning?"

"Brenda, I don't want anything to do with Mardig!"

"Okay, then why don't you use me while I'm here? I'm here now, ready to help."

"Brenda, I'm busy right now."

"Well, when would you like to get together?"

"Brenda, I have things to do. I can't drop everything every time you fly into town!"

I was trying desperately to keep my cool, but I had my fill of her diversionary ploys. "Well, you did say we would get together when I came into town! I'm in town."

"Not now!"

"Okay, when?"

"Brenda . . ."

My mind raced. Should I get angry with her or still try to hold my tongue? *"Yes, we'll get together,"* she'd say and then she'd back out. I was *sick and tired of all these excuses. For years, I watched her selfishness. I was boiling!* I let her have it. "You know what? I watch you and you can't make any commitments. You make promises and then you back out of them. You are selfish. You always have been. I'm here right now, willing to help. But all you have are excuses!" Without waiting for her reply, I hung up. *I hate doing this. It's such an immature thing to do, to slam down the phone without acknowledging the end of a conversation.*

Advice! I need advice! I e-mailed Sally. She suggested I hire an attorney to send my sister a letter inviting her to be involved. This way, the letter would be on record, as would her lack of involvement. This was a precaution since I didn't know what to expect of my family, especially if we had to go to court for anything.

Months earlier, my sister told me our brother was considering having Mardig committed. I didn't like the sound of this. Mardig and he did not get along very well. There was always the potential of a major blowup. Possibly due to Mardig's tact and diplomacy, their uneasy relationship never got out of control. *At least, this is what I saw.*

My sister and brother were nowhere to be found when there was work to be done. And when the work was finished, they were first to judge the outcome. It was better to be safe than sorry. *How do I find an attorney?*

I called the Department of Aging representative on Friday and left an urgent message requesting a list of attorneys. Saturday started the Labor Day holiday weekend, and I wanted to get this taken care of before everyone was off work until Tuesday.

Meanwhile, I continued asking Mardig to consider moving into an assisted-living community. Even though I painted idyllic pictures of living there, he didn't want to think about it until he "finished all of his work." Occasionally, however, he warmed up to the idea of being taken care of. During one of those moments, I called David and asked him to fly in for the extended holiday weekend. I wanted to accomplish *something* during this visit. David might be able to talk some sense into Mardig. After all, my chauvinistic father respected David because he is a *man*!

David flew into Milwaukee. After meeting him at the airport we drove to my father's house. Mardig enjoys David's company. Once they start talking about tools, machines, politics, or whatever, it is a while before they stop. The funny thing is, my father was unaware David had left Milwaukee in March. As far as he was concerned, David was living in the neighborhood.

While they visited, I went to the basement. I was trying to figure out what was causing an unusual odor. Was it mildew or something else? *I bet it's gas! No, it can't be. I smelled this in March!* I'll ask David. Meanwhile, I wanted to take some time to reminisce about my childhood.

In the room straight ahead was my brother's desk, where he used to study in relative quiet away from his two younger sisters, who studied and played upstairs. At my mother's insistence, he'd help me with math, algebra, and geometry. I enjoyed my brother when he was in a good mood. In fact, at times, he was a lot of fun and was quite strong. I am almost certain he could lift me off the ground as I held onto his index finger!

To the right was my father's workroom, where he kept all of his tools. On the weekends, I'd run down to see how I could help him. He worked on interesting projects and he was pleasant to be around. Mardig was patient and he would hum old tunes from the forties. When he was in a particularly cheerful mood, he would sing. My mother would say, "He doesn't know the words. He sings the same thing over and over again." Mardig rarely remembered verses, and sang only the refrains.

One day, when I was about nine years old, he entrusted me with a blowtorch. Mardig was using the soldering iron and told me I could hold the torch if I promised to pay attention. Excited, I promised. But, try as hard as I might, my mind wandered. The next thing I heard was, "Please move the torch." He said it with such self-control, I didn't pay attention. By the time he repeated it, I realized what I had done. I had burned his fingers! I was horrified and laughed nervously! He didn't get mad at me. He simply reminded me, "If you want the job, you need to keep your head about you."

I returned upstairs. David and my father were reading in the sunroom. I asked David to come to the basement with me.

"Do you smell anything?"

"Yeah, the musty odor I smell every time I come down here," he said.

"I think it's gas."

"No, it's not. It can't be."

I didn't respond.

"The whole house would have burned down if it was gas. It's musty because your father washes up and shaves down here. This is where they wash their clothes. They keep this place so closed up, it wouldn't surprise me if there is mold down here."

"David, look at Mardig. He hasn't shaved in a while. And I'm almost certain he hasn't washed any clothes!"

"I bet your brother does his laundry down here."

"Well, I think it's a gas leak. Remember, you didn't smell the leak in our home and the gas company rep found several leaks?"

"Well, call the gas company, then!"

We went upstairs and I got the telephone book to look up the number. When I explained the situation, the gas company represent-ative became concerned and said he'd have someone come over *immediately*. Sure enough, someone arrived within a couple of hours. I told him how long we had smelled this odor. As he ran his detector along the plumbing in the basement, he started to look extremely concerned.

"You have a major gas leak!"

It was a good thing Mardig and my brother didn't smoke. A flame or even a spark could have blown the whole place sky high! *The real shock was when we learned Mardig's house insurance had lapsed due to nonpayment.*

It took five workers one entire day to tear up the outside brickwork in front of the house in order to access and then seal the leaking underground valve and gas line. *Wasn't my brother taking care of the house he lived in?*

This was one of many incidents that put David and me on a mission to help Mardig. The gas leak and the empty refrigerator were evi-dence of neglect. We couldn't turn our backs on him. We had to do something. We began with simple things, like cleaning him up. The following evening, when Mardig grew weary and removed his clothes to go to bed, I grabbed the clothes he had not washed since March and washed them. I wanted to throw them away, but I feared annoying him and losing his trust.

We continued trying to get in touch with my brother. He had to be made aware of this major gas leak. He did not return our calls or the faxes we sent to his office. We didn't know how else to contact him since we had not seen him at home.

While clearing some piles of papers near one of the living room bookshelves, we found a magazine with a woman's name on it. I rec-ognized the name as the one my mother mentioned when talking about my brother's girlfriend. We decided to follow this lead. The address was in a western suburb near my brother's business. The following day we drove there to track down my brother.

We found the apartment manager who said the woman moved out months earlier. Temporarily discouraged, we went to the apartment and talked with a neighbor. The neighbor thought she had moved to Florida.

We needed information. I didn't know much about my father's affairs. How could we help him when we knew so little about this private man? Up until this point, I had not delved into Mardig's paperwork because he might react negatively to the intrusion. Things were different now; I needed to learn about his private affairs. I decided to approach it forthright and honestly. "Mardig, do you mind if I look through your files? I'd really hate for something to happen to you and then have to go through these after you're gone."

"I'm not going anywhere."

"I, ugh, well, I mean after you're gone," I stammered. "You know, dead."

Did I say that?

He looked at me and laughed. "Do you know something I don't? I plan on being around for a long time! Go ahead," he said. "I've been wanting to go through those files myself!"

"All right," I said, surprised. "We'll do it together!"

CHAPTER 4

Our Lives Take
an Unexpected Turn

D avid and I spent the next few days sorting through Mardig's papers. Mardig enjoyed our genuine interest and began reflecting on events from his earlier years. His past was a mystery to us since he did not talk about his family. Old family conflicts and misunderstandings had kept his side of the family away from ours. His mother lived her final years with his half-brother in the Chicago area. After the relationship soured between my parents and my aunt and uncle, we no longer visited them. Regrettably, my grandmother died before I had the opportunity to learn about my father's childhood.

While looking through one of the file cabinet drawers, I came upon a tattered oversized envelope. Inside was a worn brown composition book dated 1929. It was Mardig's composition book from an adult evening class to improve his English. Inside were pages filled with selected events from his childhood. I focused on an autobiographical assignment.

∞

At the tender age of five, Mardig and his mother narrowly missed the first genocide of the twentieth century. They left Van (in Turkey) just in time for the relative safety of Constantinople (now Istanbul).

I showed my father his brown composition book and asked him to read the autobiography and he recounted some of the stories of when he and a friend went swimming in the sea. David asked him about the journey coming to America in 1920 on the steamship *Pannonia* from Patras, a port in Greece. He chuckled and recounted a few stories of running around the ship and scaring his mom who was trying to keep from being seasick. When we asked about his father, Mardig changed the subject.

Curious to fill in more details, I later questioned my aunts, uncles, second and third cousins, and even my mother's side of the family. I was sickened to learn my grandfather was not *missing-in-action*, but was shot at point-blank range by a Turkish soldier. My grandfather, initially trusted and valued by the Turkish Army, was discarded once he outlived his usefulness. The last time my father saw his father was in 1918.

One-and-a-half million Armenians were tortured and mutilated during the Armenian Genocide. Stripped of their possessions, clothes, food, and water, many were murdered or left to die of thirst and starvation after being marched into the searing heat of the Syrian Desert. Others were raped and mutilated, their body parts worn as trophies by some Turkish soldiers. It's no wonder my father never spoke of his early years.

In 2002, I visited Armenia. I went to the Genocide Museum. Inside were many wall-sized photos. One was of Van, a prosperous Armenian town in the Ottoman Empire before the Turks swept through. Next to it was a photo of Van after the annihilation, not unlike the devastation to Hiroshima in World War II. *But this was 1915! How could it be this bad? The atom bomb would not be invented for another thirty years!* For the first time, tears filled my eyes as I came to the stark realization my own existence was due to the timely escape of my grandmother and father.

David and I pored through Mardig's papers. It was nearly impossible to determine what was important and what was not. We had to leaf through it all, one page at a time, being careful not to overlook something—like a $1,000 U.S. Savings Bond tucked between two sheets of scrap paper or hiding in a one-and-a-half foot pile of newspapers my brother threatened to throw away. Despite mustering some energy after discovering more details of my family history, this overwhelming task soon exhausted David and me.

After lunch one day, having washed the dishes and wiped off the table, I returned to the sunroom. I watched my father, who was hunched over paperwork in his preferred place of work and rest (there was also a bed in the room). Five arched windows lined three brick walls. Once framed by silk-lined drapes tied back to let the sun stream in, these *same* drapes, now rotted from fifty years of sun damage, were closed. A single light bulb on Mardig's desk illuminated one corner of this otherwise dark room.

I walked closer to look over his shoulder. He was organizing his bills. I sat in a chair by a bookshelf in the living room, only a few feet away from where he was working.

Soon, I grew bored and turned my attention to the books in this last of the three built-in dark oak bookshelves that lined the north wall of the living room. Some were my father's German-language books from his bachelor years; others were reference books he used for his work as a machinist. Two hardcover books covered with brown paper bags grabbed my attention. I tried to decipher the rubber-stamped letters on their spines. Reaching out, I pulled one off the bookshelf. A little package fell onto the floor. After looking quickly at the book, an engineering manual of interest to my father, brother, or David, I placed it back and reached down for the package.

Three dried-out rubber bands bound an eight-and-a-half by three-

and-a-half-inch package. I scraped off the rubber bands and unfolded a letter-sized sheet that was protecting a stack of cards. When I turned them over to look at the front side, in the upper right corner I saw "1,000" and on the upper left side "1,000." I looked at the card more carefully and read, "Series E." It finally dawned on me—it was a thousand dollar U.S. Savings Bond! I lifted a corner of the first bond to look at the second card and saw the same writing. I lifted the second bond and saw yet another "1,000." I fanned them out like a deck of playing cards and counted, four thousand, five thousand, six . . . fifteen thousand . . . twenty thousand . . . twenty-five thousand . . . twenty-eight thousand dollars in U.S. Savings Bonds. My heart fluttered!

"Mardig, look what I found!"

Without even looking up, he extended his arm and said, "Oh, give it to me. I'll look at it later." I stood up while wrapping the paper around the bonds and handed the package to him. He tossed the loosely wrapped stack of bonds on the upper right corner of his desk and then immediately placed the bill he was looking at on top. I sat down again and recalled David's comment about my father saying, "I'll look at it later."

While David was in Milwaukee during the previous year-and-a-half, he helped my father. He watched helplessly as Mardig set aside bills and other important documents until he could no longer find them. *Everything would be looked at later. Decisions would be made later.*

I decided to retrieve the savings bonds. I rose from the chair and approached my father's desk. As I reached to grab the bonds, he looked at me and asked, "What are you doing?" I pulled out the package and showed him one of the bonds.

Still showing no interest, he placed the package in the drawer. "I'll look at it later."

I was on a mission. *I had to get those bonds.*

A while later, David came into the sunroom to see what we were doing. I told him we needed to think about what we were going to eat for dinner. He exclaimed, "We just ate!"

I emphasized, "But we need to *plan* what we want to make for *dinner!*" and motioned with my head toward the kitchen. He got my hint and we went into the kitchen. I hurriedly told him about the bonds. We worked up a plan to retrieve them.

Returning to the sunroom, David distracted my father with questions about the papers on the bed. Mardig swiveled around and wheeled his chair toward his bed. With his back to the desk drawer, I swiftly retrieved the bonds and walked back to the kitchen. This was a major risk. I considered what I had just done. *I was no better than a thief!* Trembling, I fanned through them; many were thirty years old.

David and I estimated these bonds to be worth about four times their face value. I struggled to remain calm. *Mardig had over $100,000 worth of savings bonds!* Suddenly our lives became preoccupied with the bonds. *What if we lost them?* We did not take this responsibility lightly and were extremely nervous about taking them.

With the major gas leak and now this, we became vested in my father's affairs.

Still, with the overwhelming amount of paperwork, plus the fear of holding onto all this money that wasn't even ours, David and I were stressed. No one knew we had Mardig's bonds. We decided to get away. We drove cautiously to John and Anna's house and hid them in a box in the upstairs bedroom closet and then paused a moment. *There was enough money hidden in the closet to equal the price of their home!*

Since David was only in Milwaukee for the holiday weekend, our time was limited. Tethered by those bonds in the closet, we still managed to take advantage of a Labor Day weekend celebration. A microbrewery in Milwaukee was hosting *Sprecherfest*, their version of the annual Oktoberfest celebration in Germany. We went with John and Anna. Sprecher was featuring seven different brews. We ordered samplers. Now, in California, when you ask for samplers, you are served four-ounce glasses filled with three ounces of beer, hardly enough to get your tongue wet let alone decide if you like the brew. In Milwaukee, which beer made famous, they KNOW how to give you samples, sixteen-ounce plastic cups! We ordered seven of them, *each*! Afterward, we ordered two pitchers of the brews we liked best.

Returning to our table at the far corner of the tent where the live German music was blaring, we continued drinking. In our state of heightened awareness, we began to wax philosophic about the options for my father's care.

We chose the third option.

We decided to have my father live with us!

Now we had to convince Mardig of our intentions. This was the hard part. We took it slowly. We asked him a lot of *What if* questions. "What if you were to move to California?"

He didn't think it was a good idea because he had so much work to do around the house. He said he needed money. "Where would I live?" he asked.

"You would stay with us," we said eagerly.

He didn't seem excited about our idea. Being independent, he wanted to be sure he could take care of himself. We reminded him of the bonds we found, some twenty-eight thousand dollars in face value. *We downplayed their estimated value. Earlier, when I showed him his bank statement, he didn't believe he had so much.* We also reminded Mardig he had some General Electric stock; although we did not know yet how much. We knew he had a few certificates of deposit gathering interest. We estimated he was worth a couple hundred thousand, and we told him this. He laughed.

Ultimately, David managed to have a man-to-man discussion with Mardig and succeeded in persuading him to, at the very least, *visit* us in California.

The weekend was over and David had to return to California. Before leaving, he documented all the bonds: their face value, date of purchase, and serial numbers. Fortunately, this was made easier by the paper clipped copies my father kept of his bonds.

I stayed behind to handle the details. On the first day after the holiday, I went to the post office and mailed the bonds to our California home. I sent them by registered mail, which is tracked and handled carefully at each stop. *We still did not know what we were going to do with them. We just knew we did not want to lose them.* As the days rushed forward, Mardig expressed doubts about visiting us. Only slightly deterred, I continued poring through his paperwork. I separated his financial documents and inventoried them by institution or category with descriptive comments by each heading. There were bank accounts, bonds, and stock statements. After recording a document, I showed it to Mardig. With repeated showings, he began to get an idea of what he owned. In fact, he was surprised he could have amassed this much. *So was I! We were raised frugally. I wore hand-me-downs!*

I made a deal with Mardig. I told him if he had this much money, he could easily come out to California and not worry about expenses. Actually, David and I guessed he would not add much to our expenses, except meals and clothing, since the home mortgage, utilities, and other expenses were fixed regardless of whether he stayed with us or not. Besides, I wanted to get to know him better and despite his disorientation and forgetfulness, he was still in good health. Guarding his independence, Mardig questioned what would become of him if he didn't have enough money. My assurance that he could stay with us did not allay his deep-rooted concern and need for self-sufficiency.

I was relieved when he finally agreed to come to California. I excitedly e-mailed a note to David and then to Sally and Ken.

Sally replied first. Considering the options we had discussed with her earlier, we surprised her with our alcohol-induced decision. Here's an excerpt from her e-mail to me:

WOW!!!!!!! This turn I did not expect.

OK: Are you sure, you can handle this? You will be questioning every move you make from now on. You are your father's parent. You have a lot to do . . . I am in total shock; I just didn't expect this. Just wanted you to know I read your message and Ken and I will be here for you and David. Lord have mercy . . . If you need the van to pick up you and your dad at the airport just let us know … I believe in you, you'll do just fine.

Love, Sally

Usually when I return to Milwaukee, I visit friends and drive down to the Chicago area to see my aunt and uncle. *After my mother died, Mardig reestablished relations with his stepbrother. I accompanied him on several visits when I was in town. I liked being reacquainted with my family after so many years of separation.* This time I also planned to conduct a little business. Everything changed. There would be no time.

So far, I had not contacted my brother. My sister and I were no longer talking after I hung up the telephone abruptly. I was on my own. I had all of Mardig's affairs to wrap up and get him ready to move to California. *What do you take on the plane? He has a lot of things he likes: his tools, familiar clothes, grooming supplies, and paperwork. Where do I begin? What's enough? What will happen to the house?*

I was overwhelmed. There were many loose ends to tie up. And Mardig started changing his mind about accompanying me to California. *Oh, I still need to buy the plane ticket!* I had to follow up on the POA. Who would I call? I waited to hear from the Department of Aging representative who had the list. She called Tuesday afternoon. I went to her office to pick up the list and immediately called some of the attorneys. Before the end of the day, my father had an attorney who would draft his POA. Only one week remained before I returned home.

What am I doing? Is this really a smart thing to do, bringing my father to California? Am I doing something wrong? The wretched fear of the youngest child, whose parents tried to make her behave more like her older siblings, cast a long shadow. Even though my sister, brother, and I were not communicating, this was also their father I was relocating.

Feeling these doubts, I especially wanted Mardig to authorize legally my efforts to help him. I was uncertain how my brother and sister would react. I certainly didn't want them to accuse me of kidnapping our father. If I were going to take care of Mardig's affairs, I needed to do it *right*.

The attorney and I talked several times as I described the circumstances and how little time we had. He agreed to draft a document we could look at on Thursday afternoon.

Mardig still had not showered since last March. He could not go out in public this way. He was dirty and he smelled. How was I going to get him to take a shower?

On Thursday, the day we were to meet with the attorney, I used the best line of reasoning I could. Since Mardig kept telling me how much he appreciated my help, I explained that if he wanted me to take care of his affairs we would have to do it legally, meaning we had to see an attorney. "Mardig, I would feel really uncomfortable meeting with an attorney when you smell so bad."

"Do I really smell bad?" he asked, genuinely curious.

"Yes." *He encouraged candor, while he tried being the diplomat. He was a rational man and rarely got offended when he knew my comments reflected concern for his welfare.*

He surprised me when he said, "For you, I will. Now, we need to get me some clean clothes."

I laughed at his expression and assured him if he would start his shower, I would gather his clothes and have them ready for him. "Okay," he said, and went upstairs to take his shower. Just then, the phone rang. It was the attorney with some last-minute questions about the POA. He wanted to have the document ready when we arrived. As I hung up the phone, Mardig walked through the French doors into the living room wearing only a loosely buttoned shirt, no pants, and no underwear. Shocked, I averted my glance, "Why aren't you upstairs taking your shower?"

"Because you said you'd bring me some clean clothes."

"I *will*. Please go up and take your shower." I had never before seen my father even partially naked. This felt strange. "Please, Mardig. *Go upstairs*," I emphasized. "Please, take your shower."

He walked toward me and stood uncomfortably close. I feared what he might do next. "I feel very close to you right now. I know you are trying to take care of me. I love you." He then reached out to hug me. I stepped back.

My heart missed a beat or two, and I felt flush with embarrassment.

How should I respond to his appreciation and affection as he stood too close and tried to hug me with only a shirt that did a poor job covering his private parts? I had to get him upstairs to take his shower. We were scheduled to meet with the attorney and we didn't have much time. I took his hand, and trying to look away, asked him to come upstairs with me. "Remember, Mardig. You need to take a shower."

"Can you help me?" he asked.

I hesitated, and then a voice inside of me said, "If you want him to shower, just help him. It took you six months to get him to this point!" I turned my back to him as he undressed and turned on the water. *I wonder if he forgot how to use the shower after all these months.* I tried to focus only on the water and the faucet. Once the water was warm, I assisted him into the shower, taking great care to keep my eyes focused on his feet stepping over the rim of the tub. I didn't want him to trip. I closed the shower curtain and told him I would be leaving the bathroom.

Phew! That was weird! I had never had such an experience!

I went downstairs to find some clothes. He had many nice clothes, but he no longer wore them. I quietly entered the bathroom while he was still showering, and placed his clothes on the closed toilet seat and on the radiator. After he finished his shower, he called me. I walked over to the bathroom door. "Yea-us?" I hesitated, standing on the other side of the closed door.

"How do I look?" he asked.

Not knowing what to expect, I slowly opened the door and peered in through the small opening. I breathed a sigh of relief. Mardig was sitting on the toilet seat putting on his socks. He was wearing his undershirt and boxers. I opened the door completely and stepped in to look at him. Wow, he looked so clean and smelled nice. I was proud of him.

What happened moments earlier lingered in my mind.

On the way to the attorney's office, only a mile away, fear crept in. I was scared. *What should I expect?* This was such a grown-up thing to do. I was about to sign legal documents to handle my father's affairs. He had been so very private; I knew little except for the details he had shared over the last several years and the papers I had found during the past week.

We arrived at the attorney's office, located on the second floor of a neighborhood bank on the south side of Milwaukee. I turned to Mardig and exclaimed, "Race you!"

We ran up the stairs skipping every other step. *He* won! My father is in good shape, and he is forty-nine years my senior!

Breathing hard, we took our time walking down a poorly lit hallway until we found the door to the attorney's office. We opened it and a receptionist greeted us. We introduced ourselves. "Attorney Cohn is expecting you," she said.

Feeling welcome, we accepted her invitation to sit down. We barely had enough time to look around the office suite, with its solid wood paneling and tall ceilings characteristic of Milwaukee's older buildings, when Attorney Cohn appeared and introduced himself. We followed him into his office and then he shook our hands warmly, expressing his pleasure to finally meet us. He offered us two chairs in front of his desk. My father allowed me to step through the narrow space to be seated first, and then he sat down to my right. I was nervous, even with Mardig sitting next to me. This was a serious responsibility.

I looked around at the mounds of paperwork, files, and books on bookshelves, on top of the file cabinets, on the desk and credenza, and all around us on the floor. *All this paperwork! I thought I had a lot of paperwork to process.* A touch of pity vied for attention despite my nervousness. *Poor attorney! How would he get through all this paperwork?* Attorney Cohn had already drafted two powers of attorney. Only the details needed to be reviewed. I gave him credit for his efficiency! My uneasiness surfaced and I couldn't shake it.

This was an entirely new experience and I had no idea what I was getting myself into.

Attorney Cohn must have sensed my discomfort. He tried to put me at ease with his very dry humor. He was in his late forties, wore rimless glasses, and had locks of lightly salt-and-peppered curly hair. He sported a colorful pair of suspenders and a bold, bright necktie. Contrasting his vibrant accessories was a starched pima-cotton shirt, giving him the air of a true professional. It was almost as if one foot was firmly implanted in The Sixties and the other, in The Nineties. His disarming style and offer to have us address him by his first name, David, helped me to relax a little, dampening my uncertainties.

David turned to Mardig and asked him questions about his intentions. "Do you know why you are here?"

"Yes, to have my daughter manage my affairs."

"Is this your daughter?"

"Yes, this is my daughter." Mardig proudly beamed and turned to smile at me.

"What's her name?"

"Brenda."

"Can you please review these documents and let me know if you have any questions? I'll explain some of the parts to you."

Mardig didn't want to read all the pages and handed the documents to me, jokingly explaining, "You read this, since you are now managing my affairs."

What if I were doing the wrong thing? My head kept telling me to grow up and get through this. I ignored what my body was telling me. Don't do it! It's more trouble than you can possibly imagine! *Don't do it! It will turn your life upside down! Don't do it! It will totally change the course of your life!*

I insisted Mardig look through the General Durable Power of Attorney with me. I didn't understand everything. In fact, I'm not certain I read the entire document. I asked a few questions and then David drew our attention to other important parts of the document. We then spent considerable time going over the Durable Power of Attorney for Health Care. Mardig asked if I thought they were acceptable. Still nervous and with mixed emotions, I said, "Yes." I signed them and so did my father. *After all, Attorney Cohn was on the list provided by the Department of Aging. He had to be competent.*

David then asked Mardig if he understood what he had just signed.

"Yes, my daughter is my attorney!" he replied, smiling at me and patting my knee.

This step was behind us. What's next? My feelings of being overwhelmed began to suffocate me.

We went grocery shopping. Mardig had eaten most of the food we bought earlier. While we walked along the aisles, I noticed he was buoyant. He seemed childish and playful. I asked Mardig how he felt, and he said he was really happy. "You're going to help me. You really care for me." His words gave me a warm feeling. "I love you," he said. I liked hearing this, especially when he was fully dressed. *That shower incident was weird.* Then he said loudly, "I love you so much, I want to *eat* you!"

I felt embarrassed. He said it a few more times, then I asked him to stop because I was feeling embarrassed.

"Okay."

It was as if a major weight had been lifted off him. He had relinquished control. I wasn't sure how I felt about this. On the one hand, I was honored. On the other, I accepted a great responsibility. This scared me, especially since everything had happened so fast!

I called Sally about the shower incident. I was losing sleep over it. My mind *understood* Mardig's confusion, but my heart felt the opposite. I felt dirty, almost as if I'd been raped. Yet, this was too severe a feeling for what occurred, especially because my father never touched me. Still, I couldn't stop the feeling I had been violated in some way. Sally shared her experiences helping her incontinent father with toileting and then cleaning him. She explained how she tries to separate her *father* from the *man* who depends upon her for his basic daily activities. We talked long-distance for forty-five minutes. Being the youngest of three children and never babysitting, I was experiencing things others may have dealt with better. The call was a good investment. Sally helped me feel better and much stronger about helping my father in these awkward moments.

Still, the image of my father in the living room exposing himself lingered.

Armed with a POA, I could now go to the clinic and retrieve Mardig's medical records.

A few days later, I sent Sally the following e-mail of my progress.

> It has been very difficult with my father. I am trying to move much more quickly than he is comfortable. When I return Tuesday, the 10th, I hope to have him with me!
>
> David and I are trying to take this one step at a time. It's like adopting a child. Everything in our lives will change. We can't come and go as freely as we have. And we need to form proper eating habits so my father can have regular and nutritious meals! As it is, David and I lead such a hectic pace; we only eat once a day! We'll even have to get someone to care for him when both David and I are away. Since he'll be in a strange and unfamiliar place, we'd hate to see him wander and get lost! Oh well, one step at a time!

Next, I called Midwest Express Airlines and bought Mardig a *one-way* plane ticket.

It was Tuesday morning, September 10, the last day I'd be in Milwaukee. I woke up early to see John and Anna one more time before they left for work. I then showered, packed, read, and sent a few e-mails before leaving for Mardig's house.

I sent an e-mail to a business associate to explain why we were unable to meet. The following is an excerpt:

> . . . imagine getting a man who's lived in the same house for 45 years to move to Los Angeles on such short notice. I've had to, in this

brief time (one week), find a local attorney, get a power of attorney, locate and speak with my father's doctor, obtain copies of my father's medical records, take care of him day-to-day given the soon-to-be upheaval of his life . . . in short, I've managed to get by on 4 - 5 hours of sleep and take care of his affairs the rest of the time.

Everything was coming together; yet I was afraid that after all these hours of work and exhaustion from lack of sleep, I would now run into my sister and brother. I imagined a confrontation something like this:

"What? You're taking Mardig to California? WHO says?"

"Well-uh, Mardig finally said he'd come with me."

"Oh he did, did he? Mardig, do you want to go to California?"

"Uhh, no. I have so much work to do around the house. Not really. At least, not yet."

"Well, there you have it, then! Mardig doesn't want to go! You know we have laws in Wisconsin against kidnapping!"

"Well-uh, yeah, that's why we got a power of attorney."

"You got what? You saw an attorney? Behind our backs?"

I didn't want to see them now. I didn't want to fight. I was tired and running on adrenaline. I raced around the house. *What do I bring with us? He has so much stuff! His tools? There are too many! What about his stuff in the garage? Sigh!* I came to Milwaukee with only carry-on luggage, so there was no room in my bag. How would I carry Mardig's things? There were two pieces of dried-out leather-trimmed luggage in the attic. They had to be fifty years old. Those wouldn't work. A paper sack would be awkward to handle. I decided to be like a runaway child. I went upstairs to the linen closet, skipping every other stair in my hurry. Inside were my mother's old pillowcases. She had a variety and some had never been used. I grabbed one of the thick cotton ones used to cover down pillows so the feathers can't poke out. Skipping every other stair, I raced down two flights of stairs to the basement, where Mardig sometimes changed his clothes.

I packed things he would need: his wing-tipped shoes, two shirts, a pair of pants, and the new boxer shorts and undershirts we just bought.

After he agreed to come to California, we went clothes shopping. This was such an ordeal; I hope never to walk in that store again.

I gave him a pair of pants to try on. While he tried on the pants in the dressing room, I walked among the racks to look at other clothes. Out of the corner of my eye, I spotted him walking among the racks in the store in his underwear! Quickly ushering him back to the dressing room, I asked him to wait in the room, while I looked for more clothes. He complained the pants were tight around his waist. As I retrieved a larger size, I saw him among the racks; again in his underwear! I grabbed his arm this time and forcibly escorted him to the dressing area while trying to discreetly look around the store to see who saw us.

Feeling flushed, I admonished him to remain in the room, because it was embarrassing for both of us when he walked around in his worn-out underwear. His face brightened and he thanked me for looking out for him.

I headed back to the racks for more clothes. Quickly selecting another pair of pants and some shirts, I headed back when I saw him! Looking around I noticed the sales personnel were also looking while keeping their distance. I felt so embarrassed. I wished more people were aware of dementia and sensitized to what it does to a human being. After all, I could have waited with him near the dressing room while the salesperson got my father some clothes. It was a good thing we went shopping on a weekday, as the store was nearly empty.

After an hour-and-a-half of this kind of stress and his confusion, I hurriedly signed the credit card receipt for his respectable wardrobe. Mardig had new pants, shirts, pajamas, socks, and underwear.

I went to his workbench in the basement to see if there was anything else I should bring. I grabbed a magnifying glass and a tiny gray meter from the top of his workbench. I remembered the meter from my childhood; although, I wasn't sure what it was used for. At least it was small enough to bring along and he could tinker with it while in California.

I ran upstairs, skipping steps again. I had to hurry! I didn't want to run into my brother or sister. In the sunroom, I found another magnifying glass. I pulled the first one out and noticed there was a slight difference between the two. One was a solid piece of glass held by a metal band mounted on a plastic handle and the other was entirely plastic with a tiny higher-powered magnification embedded in the larger portion of the lens. I put them both in the pillowcase and then picked up a pair of Mardig's glasses. He seemed to alternate between two pairs. I opened his desk drawers and grabbed his wallet, an envelope with some cash, and a few bank statements that I rolled up and tucked among his clothes in the bag. I also found a little brown jewelry box. This contained his hearing aid. *Why wasn't he wearing it?* I found another pair of glasses, adding them to the collection. I placed the two powers of attorney in the pillowcase and was ready to go.

At about 7:00 p.m., as the sun was setting in Milwaukee, my father and I boarded a plane for Los Angeles. This was his first commercial flight. Sitting by the window, Mardig couldn't fathom the idea of flying six to seven miles above the ground. He also couldn't imagine such a good meal being served on a plane. In fact, he didn't believe he was *flying in a plane*.

He refused to believe me when I told him how high we were flying, so he got up to ask the flight attendants. I watched him as he talked and laughed with the flight attendants at the front of the plane. Perhaps they relished Mardig's innocence and genuine kindness; they entertained him for nearly an hour. When he returned to his seat, he had been given his *wings*—a tradition where a flight attendant or sometimes the pilot will pin wings on a person's chest during their *first* flight. Usually reserved for children, my father had to be the oldest *child* who *earned* his wings at age eighty-six.

Two

A Grain of Sand

Mardig had been with us awhile and David and I spent any spare time we had on his affairs. We grew increasingly frustrated and began to spiral into hopelessness. Each time we thought we were making progress, there was more. We stayed awake at night, churning details in our minds, making sure we hadn't forgotten anything and had considered our options. Even so, we could not foresee the magnitude of the responsibility we had undertaken.

In less than fourteen days, our lives dramatically changed. Caregivers and professionals comforted us with their assessments. "What you accomplished in two weeks usually takes several months to a year!"

I called Mardig's attorney to complain. David Cohn put it into perspective with two simple analogies: "You decided to pick up an acorn and instead got the whole oak tree! You decided to pick up a grain of sand and instead got the whole beach!"

I laughed when he said this and, in the following months, I actually visualized the long, wide sandy beaches along the California coast. I realized the vast difference between picking up one grain of sand and being stuck with the whole beach!

This actually helped me feel better.

CHAPTER 5

We Become Parents

O nce we landed in Los Angeles, Mardig was happy to see David. He and David talked for an hour-and-a-half on the drive home. I closed my eyes and fell into a light sleep in the backseat of the car. I was exhausted.

At 11:00 p.m. Pacific Time, after a six-hour trip (four-hour flight and two hours including the drive home), my father walked into our home and looked around. *David had taken great care to prepare Mardig's room and bathroom. He bought things Mardig needed: toiletries, more underwear than the few I had bought in Milwaukee, and food for healthy and balanced meals.* Mardig would have none of it. Disoriented, he insisted on going home. He pledged to visit us the following day, but for now, he needed to return home for the night.

What are we going to do? We explained how far he had traveled. It took us another hour-and-a-half to persuade Mardig to spend the night. We promised to take him home in the morning. *What began as a caring gesture on our part, with months of preparation and two intense weeks of labor, would be shortened by Mardig's insistence on returning home. If he really wanted to return to Milwaukee, we would fly back with him the following day.*

The next morning, he awoke well rested. David had taken the day off from work and was making breakfast when I came into the kitchen. After months of eating only one balanced meal every weekday from the home delivered meals program, Mardig was delighted to sit down to a hearty breakfast of eggs, bread, cheese, and grapefruit. *So were we! We rarely ate breakfast. But we had to change our routine. We were responsible for Mardig now.*

After breakfast, I asked Mardig to come with me for a short drive around the neighborhood. I wasn't convinced he knew where he was, so I wanted him to see the area in the daylight. Also, I wanted him to feel free to confide in me privately if he needed to.

Like a child becoming aware of the world around him, he commented about everything he saw—the newer homes with their red tile roofs; the clean, wide streets; and the tall, narrow cypress trees. In contrast, I was still tired from the intensely stressful journey to get him to California and I was tense due to the amount of work that I knew had accumulated in my absence. We returned home. Mardig started asking many questions. Feeling distracted by my work, I asked David to spend time with Mardig. David offered to occupy him.

"Mardig, would you like to take a walk with me?" David asked my father, who had followed me into my home office.

Like an excited child, Mardig said, "Yes!"

He loved to walk and we hoped it would help him become familiar with his new surroundings. They put on their shoes and left for what David assured me would be a forty-five minute walk. *Ahhh. Peace. Quiet. Relaxation.*

Exhausted, I struggled to keep my heavy eyelids open. I sat at my desk, playing tug-of-war in my mind. *Should I take a nap or make a dent in my work?*

I had not heard from my sister since that ill-fated telephone call, so I phoned and left a message. I also sent her an e-mail, knowing she would at least read a note from me. I felt uncomfortable with her not being involved. Trying to appear upbeat, I wrote:

Subject: MARDIG
Hi!

Hey, I left a message on your answering machine . . . it was shortly before 1:00 p.m. your time.

I managed to persuade Mardig to come to California with me. The logistics were no easy feat! Taking a man on his first commercial airline flight and leaving his home of 45 years. By the way, he earned his WINGS. The flight attendants pinned them on his jacket!

I bought him clothes (you know how dirty and worn his clothes were) pants, shirts, PJs, underwear, and socks and got him to take a shower (after five months without one?). Actually, I wish you could have seen him, HE LOOKS PRETTY COOL!

So, he's here and I'm one tired puppy! He really needs a lot of looking after . . . especially since he is in unfamiliar territory. I took him for a drive and then David went with him for a walk.

Well, this is all I will share with you for now. Hope his being out here provides you a brief respite. By the way, I haven't reached [our brother] yet . . . his reaction should be interesting.

Tryin' to do what I can for Mardig,
Brenda

I knew David and I were going to take this journey without any support from my sister or brother, so I reached out to my friends and colleagues, soliciting their advice mostly by e-mail. This way, they could read their messages when it was convenient for them. They wouldn't have to endure long-winded telephone conversations begging for advice, understanding, pity, compassion, or sympathy. One of my e-mails was to a colleague who had moved to San Diego. I had promised to visit him in his new home once I returned to California.

Subject: HELLO FROM CALIFORNIA!
Rodger,

Helloooooo . . . I'm Baaaaack! Uh-ohhh.

Update: I have brought my father out here to live with David and me. So, this'll put a little different spin on things—freedom, accessibility, sleep (he wanders at night) . . . David and I take turns getting up and taking twenty minutes or so to talk him into going back to sleep. Hey, it's like havin' a BABY!

Once things settle a little bit then we'll see how I can work out a trip to your neck o' the woods (oops, beach!). I'll bring you a cigar. (It's a BOY!)

I hope you are settling in nicely and that you've been at a beer race already!

> Brenda Avadian
> Speaker, Author, & Human Development Consultant

During breakfast one weekend morning, Mardig shared his appreciation for our care and wanted to know why we were going out of our way for him. I told him because he was my father and reminded him of the power of attorney. He smiled at the idea we would care for him *simply* because he was my father. He then asked if I had the POA papers. I said, "Yes," and went into his room to get the papers for him. He read them quietly for about thirty minutes while David and I cleared off the table and washed the dishes.

"The person who wrote this is not *just* an attorney, but *an attorney*!" Mardig blurted out. He then asked, "So, I've appointed you to take care of *every*thing?" emphasizing the word *every*.

"Yes," I replied hesitatingly, unsure where his comments were leading.

"Good," he said, much to my relief. "Now I don't have to worry about *any*thing!"

I sent an e-mail to David Cohn to update him on how Mardig was doing in California, and to give him my father's feedback on the POA he had authored. I still had not heard from my sister or brother, and asked him to follow up on determining who owned the home Mardig just vacated. *My brother had repeatedly told my sister our father's house was his (my brother's). We needed to be sure who the owner was.*

Later, Mardig brought up the subject of his finances. "Okay, we have an account in Omaha. We need to get that money." *He meant, we need to get in the car and drive to Nebraska!*

"All right, we'll do that," I half-heartedly replied. There was a lot to do before we could grasp the entirety of his affairs. *When will I ever get my own work done?*

∽

During the following weeks, I made many phone calls and sent and received many more e-mails. I needed to let as many people know what we'd done. Their reactions helped me; especially because I started to question every move I made and, without my sister and brother's involvement, I felt uncomfortably alone.

Among the calls I made were to my neighbors. Weighing the potential embarrassment of letting neighbors know private family business versus the risk of Mardig disappearing without us being aware, I opted to tell them the truth. "David and I have adopted my eighty-six-year-old father, who was diagnosed with dementia. He's about five feet and one inch tall and weighs 112 pounds." *He lost a lot of weight in Milwaukee.* "He typically wears black-rimmed glasses, a baseball cap, and a brown jacket. If you see him on the street, please call us because he's not familiar with this area and will get lost easily."

Two days later, one of our neighbors called to say she was looking out her kitchen window and saw someone who matched Mardig's description walking toward the end of our block. David ran out to bring him back.

At the end of the month, Mardig and I went clothes shopping. He looked so nice in the new clothes we had bought earlier; I wanted to buy him more so he'd have a greater variety. Despite our Milwaukee shopping experience, I had more confidence, because now I knew what sizes he wore. We bought pants, shirts, polo shirts, socks, and underwear. He'd look like a Californian.

David was typically gone thirteen hours each day—a four-hour commute plus a nine-hour workday. In October I would have to take an out-of-town business trip. Who would care for Mardig?

Two special friends volunteered to help after some careful planning, ingenuity, and heavy reliance on my father's charm. Jan would take care of Mardig in the mornings, and Sally agreed to care for him in the evenings. Thanks to Sally, we had already arranged for the six or seven hours between when Jan and Sally would care for Mardig.

We decided to do a trial run with Jan before I left on my trip.

Sally was already caring for her father so we felt assured she could manage Mardig. Besides, Sally's husband, Ken, was available to help if necessary and a locked wrought iron fence protected their home. Mardig would not be able to wander out into the street and get lost.

Jan was in an entirely different situation. She would be the sole caregiver for Mardig after her husband, Dave, left for work at 6:15 a.m. She lived on a quarter-acre in a rural area accessed by a busy street.

At 4:30 a.m., David took Mardig to Jan's house.

Jan phoned to let me know her morning with my father had been enjoyable. I was relieved! She and my father talked, drank juice, shared a breakfast muffin, and read the paper. Mardig asked for maps wanting to know where he was.

I feel sad that my father doesn't know where he is. Everything is different here, in the high desert, compared to what he was used to in Milwaukee. We live in a vast valley surrounded by distant mountains and a 360-degree view of the horizon. Eighty miles north of Los Angeles, the Antelope Valley is dotted with Joshua trees and new housing developments. In this strange and unfamiliar place, my father drew comfort from kind and loving people. Yet, he would never realize he had achieved his and my mother's long-held dream to move to California.

Our plan worked. I was thankful Jan and Mardig enjoyed one another. He remembered her and called her "the barefoot lady." Jan rarely wore shoes or socks at home. Mardig, who couldn't remember names (I inherited this weakness), easily remembered the nickname he gave to Jan. When asked, he could even describe what she looked like and on what side of town she lived.

Likewise, Jan looked forward to Mardig's company because he was pleasant and he reminded her of her late father. One weekend, David, Mardig, and I visited Jan and Dave. It was a cool fall afternoon. David, Dave, and my father went out into the backyard to look at Dave's progress restoring his collection of old Corvettes. Jan and I stood in the kitchen, where it was warmer, and looked out the window while sipping our drinks. Suddenly Jan grabbed my forearm.

Hardly able to contain herself, she exclaimed, "Just look at him!" She pointed toward Mardig. "He looks so much like *my* father!"

One of our business partners, a good friend, and Jan's newest neighbor, recognized Jan and Mardig's special relationship in the following e-mail she sent to me while I was in Mississippi.

> Hey Girl!
> Sounds like you are having a really good time . . .
> We are planning a show on Friday . . . When you get back we need to toss over some ideas . . .
> I saw Jan one morning with your father. She was showing him the mailbox. She must be a wonderful woman. I hope to get to know her better.
> Have a good trip in the South. That's my old stomping grounds and I miss it much.
> See you on your return.

Even during my time of need to have Mardig cared for while I was traveling on business, my father was able to be a gift to Jan by reminding her of her father.

At the end of the day, Sally cared for Mardig. He read, watched TV, or looked at maps until David came two or three hours later. Sometimes when David was late (Los Angeles traffic is unpredictable), Mardig would join Sally and her family for dinner.

Wow! Special friends are truly invaluable.

It was amazing how this one addition to our lives would impact the entire fabric of our relationships with others.

One business colleague wrote: "You and David are performing a noble act." Given her experience with her uncle, she added, "It's like having a child." I replied to her e-mail:

> Thank you for your kind words. Yes, he is David's and my eighty-six-year-old son. We will give him a safe place to live his life with dignity.

We have learned to go without a full night of sleep . . . as with a child, we must get up periodically and cajole him back to sleep.

He also gets very confused when he returns after we take him out. I like him to be stimulated; yet, I can begin to see why so many elderly are placed into nursing homes and drugged into sedation. If he wasn't my father, I doubt David and I could be so patient with him. As you may suspect, we have slowed down tremendously since he's come into our lives.

Caring for Mardig would prevent me from seeing this colleague until a year later. I even stopped using my "Speaker, Author, & Consultant" signature block when sending e-mails because my time was now dominated by Mardig's affairs. Fearing loss of my identity and the business I had so carefully grown, I regrettably stopped being able to fulfill my speaking and consulting obligations.

Another colleague wrote:

David and you are extraordinary folks—not everyone can accept the work and responsibility involved in caring for an Alzheimer's relative, even a beloved member of the family. I tip my hat to you both.

Later, a former business associate and his wife, who are two of the most disciplined people I know, wrote:

Taking your father under your care will certainly be a challenge, and we commend you for your faith and concern . . . most people would not want nor be willing to make such a stretch.

They weren't kidding!

CHAPTER 6

Adult Day Care

W e are barely keeping up! We need to get Mardig quality medical care. Even though the clinic in Milwaukee did a decent job of serving his needs, we want to get him specialized care to gain greater insight into his condition. Also, his time-consuming nightmarish financial affairs need attention. *That reminds me, we need to get his bonds out of our house!*

At first, we looked for ways to keep Mardig active during the day. In Milwaukee, he was familiar with his neighborhood and walked around, shopped, did his banking, etc. Here, everything is spread out and Mardig is still unfamiliar with the area. He loves to read, so we ordered the newspaper for him. He also read magazines and books. After several days, though, he had enough. He wanted to *do* something! Even with the variety and quantity of books we had, his nearly unquenchable appetite for reading had been filled.

I looked around for things to *do*. We live in a newer home, so there are limited opportunities for him to do what he loves: fix things. We did have a couple of outdoor electrical outlets giving us some problems. I asked Mardig if he was willing to fix these. *I was taking a risk, due to his diminished capacity. But I weighed this with how useful he would feel.* He said he'd be happy to fix them and completed the work in one afternoon. This wasn't enough to keep his mind active. He needed more to do.

Mardig started looking at the classified ads for a job. I offered to help him find one. Wal-Mart hires retirees, maybe he could work there. He was warm, congenial, and personable. He would love it! I imagined him, as a greeter at Wal-Mart. He'd welcome people to the store and then wish them a good day as they left. Then one day, an attractive lady with a cart full of items would catch his eye. He'd offer to help her to her car, and once out in the parking lot, he would be disoriented and get lost! It would be the shortest job he ever had!

I brainstormed other job opportunities for him with friends and associates. In this quest, I almost overlooked Mardig's impairment. His bouts of disorientation would be a problem at any *real* job. I began to look at other options.

Sally used to take her father to the local Visiting Nurse Association's Adult Day Care (ADC)[1] Center and highly recommended it. It kept her father's mind active and allowed him to socialize. At first, I didn't like the idea. After all, parents take their *children* to day care. Children don't take *parents* to day care. At least this is what I believed. *I had so much to learn.*

Since Sally repeatedly urged me to consider day care, I called to inquire. Roberta, the administrator at the ADC answered the telephone. After explaining my situation to her, she invited me to visit.

A day later, I went to see what the center looked like. I went unannounced and Roberta was not prepared to see me. She was helping a family of one of the participants; they were arranging to remove their mother due to her declining health and need for skilled nursing care. The son and daughter-in-law were in Roberta's office exchanging teary-eyed good-byes.

While waiting, my attention was drawn to the participants. I was not prepared to see these mostly older participants treated with the same warmth and compassion one would give to a *child*. I tried to

---

1 The Visiting Nurse Association's Adult Day Care (ADC) changed ownership several times. Today, the Lancaster Adult Day Health Care Center offers socialization and is also licensed for health care.

accept this as yet another new experience, yet it was challenging to watch elderly people in a diminished state being sweet-talked, and doing activities more suited to elementary school children. I'd have to get Sally's perspective on dealing with this. *After all, my options to provide stimulating activities for my father were limited!*

I was also feeling embarrassed. *Brenda's father is going to day care. What would others think? What kind of daughter would take her father to day care? Why not let him stay at home, where she can care for him? Why give someone else the responsibility?*

And then there were those other concerns. *How could my father possibly fit in? He wasn't this bad.*

Roberta finished attending to the family and came out of her office to see me. Graciously taking time to meet me while containing her emotions, she explained the participants become family and it is hard to see them leave.

As the family walked past us to leave, Roberta excused herself and reached out to hug the participant and to say good-bye. As we watched them walk out the door, she wiped her tears and apologized for falling apart. I was moved by her genuine emotion and visualized her feeling this way about Mardig someday.

After watching this heartfelt farewell and having my questions answered, my feelings and embarrassment about bringing Mardig to the ADC started to melt away. As I watched the staff's compassion for the participants, my concerns turned into reasons to bring him here. *At least Mardig would be treated with kindness. He would be treated gently. He would receive the attention he needed; more than I, one person, could give.*

But what about customized care? Mardig couldn't go to day care. He wanted to work!

"Roberta, do you provide customized care for the participants?" I explained, "My father needs to feel useful. He needs to believe he is contributing to our household. He wants to go to work and earn money. He says he's not ready to retire."

"How old is your father?"

"Eighty-six."

Lightly laughing, she explained, "The staff treats each participant uniquely. If a participant wants to go to work, the staff greets him by welcoming him to *work* and then giving him the day's tasks to perform. If a participant thinks she's going to go to school, they welcome her to school and gave her lessons."

"You really do this?" I asked, amazed.

"Yes, of course!" Roberta replied. "Otherwise, the participants wouldn't be happy."

"You mean, you learn what each person needs and then you deal with them in that way?"

"Yes. We meet with the family and learn what each participant wants and likes. If your father wants to go to work, then each member will refer to work when talking with your father," she emphasized.

I like this personal touch!

I spent forty-five minutes at the ADC and met several of the staff members: Ellie, Tee, David, and Kathy; and a few of the participants.

Even though Mardig seemed in better shape than the participants I saw, he needed to remain active. Besides, while he was at the ADC, I would have time to run my consulting and television network businesses. I told Roberta I'd give it a try. She gave me a Participant Agreement form to complete when I brought in my father.

I went home and discussed the idea with Mardig. "This place (I did not call it by name.) is like a job. It will be your initial training before you can move into higher-level responsibilities."

He was thrilled. "I'll try it!" he said eagerly.

I filled out the form Roberta gave me.

My conscience started to bother me. For the first time since we began actively helping my father, I had outright lied to him. He was not stupid. He would see the day care for what it was and ask me why I took him to a place where they make crafts, do busywork, and take frequent breaks.

I remembered visiting my father at the neighborhood factory; he worked part-time in the mornings to earn extra income before he retired. I was between ten and thirteen years old. It was summertime, when kids looked for things to do since school was out. I would walk about a mile, sometimes alone or with my sister, to visit him. I'd wait for the bell to ring; signaling break time. When I couldn't find him, I'd look inside the dimly lit factory and be surprised to see him still working. Usually one of his co-workers would notice me and ask if I wanted to see my father. I'd eagerly nod and say, "Yes!" The worker would explain, "Oh, Marty? He's still working. He should be on break, but he just keeps working. Wait and I'll get 'im for you."

While I waited, I'd be a little afraid of how my father would react, since I was interrupting his work. Sometimes I'd just walk up to the machine he was working on and he'd look up with a big smile and say, "Oh, let me finish up. Wait for me outside and I'll come out and talk with you." (This was in the days before safety regulations impacted this factory.) He'd come out and talk with me. Then, five minutes later, before the bell rang to signal people back to work, he'd say, "I have to get back to work. Thank you for visiting. Are you going home now?" I would be disappointed he cut our visit short to return to work before break time was over. After all, I had walked quite a distance. But that's the way he was.

I told David about the lie. What would happen if Mardig saw through this charade and realized this was not a job, but just a place to socialize and stay active? He had *worked* at home. He took motors apart, cleaned the parts, and put them back together. He tried to process his paperwork and took care of his banking. He organized his tools, and even worked in the yard. David and I decided to take the chance.

We justified the benefits of having Mardig socialize and be engaged in activities. Mardig had been a hermit for way too long. During the last few months he lived in Milwaukee, Mardig spent most days at home, except when he went grocery shopping and visited the bank. Still, David also shared my concern about lying to Mardig. We slept restlessly that night. I worried about Mardig's reaction. I certainly did not want to offend him, or more importantly, to lose his trust.

The following morning Mardig showered at my urging. "You want to be clean for your first day of work." He put on the clothes I selected for him. He liked when I made a fuss over him.

"Even Ma (referring to my mother) didn't fuss over me this much!"

Well, maybe she didn't during the last years of her life, but she certainly did while he was working. He was without a doubt the cleanest and best-dressed machinist at General Electric, his full-time job starting in the afternoon. He showered twice a day and my mother made sure he had clean and pressed clothes to wear to work each day.

We had breakfast and joked about his first day at a new job. I teased him and asked him to be good; I didn't want any calls from his supervisor. He said he'd make me proud, because he knew my reputation was riding on this job referral. I was pleased he was looking forward to his new job, but it came at a price—I had lied.

I drove Mardig to *work* and the staff warmly welcomed him. A smiling staff member offered him a cup of coffee with plenty of cream and sugar. Mardig was not a coffee drinker, but he politely accepted her gesture and savored the sweet and creamy taste. With the warm reception, he was able to relax. I walked into Roberta's office and handed her the completed paperwork. She assured me there was nothing to worry about. "We'll take good care of your father," another staff member added, as I turned to leave.

I returned home to peace and uninterrupted quiet. I immediately started to work. Soon, though, worries crept in. *I wonder how Mardig's doing. What is he doing right now? Will he be mad at me for taking him there?* After a couple hours of wondering and not being able to concentrate on my work, I called the ADC. The staff member who answered the phone assured me he was doing great. She said he was a hit with the ladies. *This was a side of my father I didn't know about!* I was happy knowing he was fitting in. There was still the nagging question about what he would say when I picked him up that afternoon. Since Mardig is the master diplomat, he wouldn't say anything to people *at work*. He would wait until he saw *me*.

I drove to the ADC to bring Mardig home. He looked happy and was in a joyful mood. The staff told me they enjoyed him a lot and asked if I would bring him again.

"I'd like to bring him in tomorrow, but first I want to see how he reacts this evening to his first day of work."

On the way home, Mardig talked about how much he enjoyed what he had done. Then he added, "If *that* is called *work*, then work has changed a lot since I worked at General Electric!" *He hadn't seen through the charade!*

When David came home, Mardig said the same thing to him. We were pleased. This meant he would be around people, involved in a variety of activities, go for walks, and most importantly, be supervised by a caring staff. This also meant I would have six hours each day to accomplish my work.

For the most part, Mardig's participation in adult day care worked well. He enjoyed the staff, participants, and activities. I learned he relished dancing with the ladies. Considering there were more ladies than men, he frequently danced with different partners. Since he was in such good physical shape, he'd dance every dance, tiring his partners who were ten and twenty years his junior!

Mardig had helped care for my mother during the last decade of her life, and then lived virtually alone for the three years since her death. It thrilled me to see my well-dressed and groomed father getting attention as he enjoyed these last years of his life. He deserved it!

Each afternoon when I picked him up, the staff told me what Mardig had worked on. Sometimes, Mardig brought home a craft or art piece he had created. He wouldn't think much of it and toss it aside, but I would treasure it like a proud parent. I'd even place some of his artwork on the refrigerator door!

We were also able to arrange for Mardig to be *paid* for his work. Roberta engineered the deception by handing me an envelope every Friday with the receipt enclosed for the weekly ADC bill. It was a small price to pay for the enormous benefits. Mardig assumed this was his paycheck and that the funds went toward his expenses in our home. He never asked to see the contents.

As the weeks passed, Mardig's wandering increased at the adult day care, just as it did at home. Sometimes he moved about excessively and challenged the staff by refusing to return after walking outside. One afternoon, while I was traveling between Texas and Mississippi on business, he refused to come inside. The staff called David at work to help control Mardig. David left work immediately and drove two hours from his office to the day care center just to bring Mardig home.

The adult day care center recommended we get Mardig a Safe Return™ bracelet provided through the national Alzheimer's Association. The Safe Return™ Program provides families peace of mind by registering their loved ones in a national program collaborating with law enforcement. When I objected to the bracelet or any other item of jewelry, because my father would refuse to wear it, the staff suggested he might be more accepting if *they* gave it to him as a gift. *What a great idea!*

I completed the paperwork, paid the nominal fee, and once the bracelet arrived, placed it in a nice velvet jewelry box. The staff presented it to Mardig and he accepted their gift. The bracelet is engraved with an identifier number and a toll-free telephone number to call if the person is found. It is designed so that it's difficult to remove. Sometimes Mardig tried to take it off, but for the time being, it remained around his wrist. Given his wandering, I felt more secure knowing he had the bracelet.

The adult day care center offered other benefits toward my father's well being. He had many opportunities to socialize, to remain active, to think, to smile, to laugh, and to do all the things he deserved to do.

I took Mardig to the ADC almost five days a week. We followed a routine. After he came home, he'd get the mail and then read magazines until David came home about 6:00 p.m. We would eat dinner, talk awhile, read, or watch television. Mardig preferred to go to bed early; at about 8:30 p.m. David and I would stay up and do housework or read the rest of the mail.

I started adapting to my father's schedule. David would rise at 4:15 a.m. to make the long drive to Los Angeles. I would get up an hour later to quickly shower and then get some uninterrupted work done before my father woke up. Mardig would sometimes get up and find me in my office so that we could talk. I'd encourage him to return to bed so he would be well rested for work. Then I'd continue working until 6:30 or 7:00 a.m., when I'd go to his room to wake him.

But Mardig started to resist going back to bed after waking up early. He'd come into my home office, fully dressed and ready to *leave* for work. Each time, I tried talking him into going back to bed. He didn't.

One morning I closed the door to my office, hoping he wouldn't notice me. He didn't bother me that morning. But I couldn't get any work done either, because I tried to hear what he was doing on the other side of the closed door! I heard him pacing. I heard him open the refrigerator door, then return to his room. I got up from my chair and carefully opened the door, making sure I didn't make a noise. I peered down the hallway toward his room. Quietly, I moved toward the kitchen to check if the refrigerator door was closed tightly, something he often overlooked. Everything looked fine. There was a candy wrapper on the counter and a few pieces of candy were missing from the candy bowl.

I tiptoed toward Mardig's room so he wouldn't hear me. His door was slightly ajar. From the small opening, I saw him sitting in the rocking chair, his back turned to me. I wasn't sure whether he was sleeping or not. Curiosity got the better of me, so I slowly opened the door, unsure if it would creak and he would hear me. It didn't. Since he couldn't hear well, I was able to sneak up beside him. His eyes were closed. Three crumbled candy wrappers were on the floor and one of David's engineering books rested on his lap. On one of the bookshelves, within easy reach, was a partially filled glass of milk. Despite the urge to wake him and help him back to bed, where he would be more comfortable, I let him be, went back into my office, and closed the door.

I worried his neck and back would be sore from sleeping in the chair. He frequently slept this way and rarely complained. After a couple hours, he knocked on my office door. I stopped what I was doing to make us breakfast. We talked until it was time for me to take him to work.

I tried leaving my office door closed the next morning. It worked. I tried it again. It worked. *So far, so good.*

Many mornings, I accomplished ninety minutes of work before Mardig knocked on my office door. He was polite. He would knock before entering.

Every other morning I would help him take a shower. After my experience in Milwaukee, I approached this activity differently. Sally's comments helped me approach these showers with a healthier perspective. I knew Mardig was dependent on me. I laid out his clothes and even helped him get dressed. Then I prepared breakfast and took him to the adult day care center.

Our morning ritual; however, would not continue smoothly.

CHAPTER 7

"Where's my shoes?"[1]

David and I ask our guests to take off their shoes in the foyer before walking into our home. We think the carpet will stay cleaner, especially since we can't monitor what's being tracked in off the street. Mardig, a product of the Depression, believes a *man needs to wear his shoes.*

We bought him a pair of wool-lined suede moccasins to wear in the house. He complained each time we asked him to put them on. He preferred his heavy leather shoes with thick leather soles.

"Mardig, please don't wear your shoes in the house."

"Why?"

"Because we don't wear shoes in the house. It keeps the carpet cleaner."

"My shoes are not dirty. See?" He turns up the soles of his shoes to prove his point.

"Yes, I see. But you don't know where they've been. We like to sit or lie on the floor without worrying about germs."

Mardig wasn't worried about germs. He'd tease my mother, "A little germ won't hurt anyone," when she'd remind him to wash his hands.

---

1 Despite the incorrect grammar, this is exactly how Mardig asked the question. Thus, the book title and references to this question appear in quotation marks.

"Mardig, please take your shoes off and wear your slippers. See? They're lined with lambs wool."

"Those aren't *shoes*."

"That's right, they're *slippers*. You know, *pategs*," I emphasized in Armenian. "Please put them on."

We'd argue like this. Some days it didn't get me anywhere. My father would wear his slippers—until he spotted his shoes in his bedroom. Then he'd immediately remove the moccasins and put on his shoes. David gave up. I lost patience. David tried to convince me it was useless; and I began to feel like a bad person. I remembered my brother's irritation with Mardig when he'd forget or could not hear him. I imagined I was becoming like my brother. *This was scary!* As much as I despised his lack of patience with our father, this repeated shoe incident was helping me to empathize with him. I was growing irritated, this shoe battle was taking too much of my energy.

What's the big deal? All we need to do is get the carpets cleaned. Then I considered what's involved in getting carpets cleaned. I'd have to get quotes, set time aside to have them clean the carpets, help move the furniture, put little foil pieces under the legs of tables, chairs, dressers, couches, beds, and wait for the carpet to dry. I did not have time for this. Plus, the inconvenience would upset my father's routine and he might forget and walk on the wet carpets with his shoes. *All he had to do is wear slippers to avoid all this trouble.* I decided he was going to cooperate on this one thing!

Morning, noon, and night, I thought about how to get my father to comply. Finally, I had a plan. With David's cooperation, we would hide Mardig's shoes! After he took off his shoes before going to bed, we would hide them. We would only give him his shoes before he went outside.

When Mardig went to bed that night, we went in to say good night. I discreetly stooped down, plucked up his neatly paired shoes from under the bed, and pirouetted out of the room without his realizing what had happened.

Later, Mardig awoke, got dressed, and couldn't find his shoes. He walked into our bedroom, *"Where's my shoes?"*

"Wha . . .?" Squinting, to shield my eyes from the beam of light from his flashlight, I asked, "Why? Do you need them?"

"Yes. I'm going to work?"

"At *this* time?"

"I don't want to be late."

"You won't be. You're at least six hours early."

"I am?"

"Yes. You don't start work until eight."

"What time is it?"

"It's one-thirty in the morning."

"Oh, well then, *where's my shoes?* I don't want to be late."

Since David had a two-hour commute ahead of him in a little over three hours, I got up and walked Mardig back to his room. After a half hour and my pledge to wake him in time so he wouldn't be late for work, he undressed and went back to sleep. I returned to bed and lay awake.

Got away with that one. We didn't even have to tell him where his shoes were!

At 3:00 the next morning, I gradually awoke from a deep sleep. Mardig was in our bedroom asking, *"Where's my shoes?"* David told him he didn't know. He persuaded him to go back to bed and said he would help my father find the shoes in the morning.

In solving one problem, we had created another. Those three words would soon make our hearts race and our hairs stand on end.

This was our newest *early* morning ritual. Mardig awoke at any hour of the night and wandered the house. Many mornings, he was looking for someone. He'd finally make his way into our bedroom and wake us up while he shuffled about. We learned how to sleep lightly, just like parents who wake to their children's slightest sounds. We reminded ourselves we had made the decision to *adopt* my father and had taken on the role of parents.

Some nights he came into our bedroom and patted the walls for a light switch. We'd been surprised enough nights with a sudden bright light to finally disconnect the light from the wall switch. *Even the sun slowly rises above the horizon, gradually unveiling its bright glory each morning!*

Mardig resorted to using a flashlight more frequently. I remember as a little girl, he'd use a flashlight to walk around the house at night. He had a rubber-encased flashlight he found under the seat of a used car he'd bought for $600. Long after the car was gone, he'd tell us, "The car was free, and the flashlight was $600." When we asked to use it, he'd remind us, "Be careful, that's my $600 flashlight."

Many mornings, a light shining in our faces awakened David and me, and we immediately feared a burglar was in the house. Jolted out of an already compromised sleep, we'd realize it was Mardig. Fortunately, for us, he had taken it apart and put it together so many times, pieces were missing, and it no longer worked.

He adapted to this challenge by patting the walls, the furniture, and us! He'd feel around the bed and our bodies. If we were awake, we'd take care to hold very still and not breathe. We felt very uncomfortable and feared we might reactively jerk if he accidentally touched us in a private place. Thankfully, he never did. We hoped by ignoring him, he would go back to bed. Instead, he was scared and called out our names. Our hearts softened. We took turns getting up to comfort our *frightened child* as we cajoled him back to bed.

Sometime later, when I was exhausted, I asked Sally for help. She recommended we lock our bedroom door. Concerned, I asked, "But what about my father? Wouldn't this be too traumatic for him?" Sally reminded me that David and I were running out of energy. We were not getting enough sleep. She assured us our ears would pick up the important sounds and this may be a way to discourage Mardig from getting up at night. *She should know. She's a mother of three!*

David and I preferred to sleep with our bedroom door open. It was time for us to change our ways. We not only had to close our bedroom door, but lock it as well. We tried it. We didn't sleep well the first night. We worried how Mardig would fare. Mardig got up to go to the bathroom and then slept the rest of the night.

The second night he tried the door to our bedroom. When it didn't open, he jiggled the doorknob. When this too failed, he walked away. As we drifted back to sleep, the doorknob began to jiggle again. Throughout the night, he jiggled the doorknob, keeping us awake. We tried to lie silently, like two trembling Chihuahuas, fearing what could happen on the other side of that door.

This was the option for our sanity and rest. *But were we really getting any rest?* We heard Mardig walk toward the living room. The following morning he was sleeping on the recliner, wearing his brown jacket, pajamas, and slippers. He looked so innocent, so peaceful, like a child. I felt sorry for him. He had lost his sense of time.

On other nights, we heard the creak of the front door as he tried to leave. We have security screen doors locked with keys from both inside and outside. Mardig couldn't get out. After some time, he returned and jiggled the doorknob to our bedroom again.

One night we heard noises from the utility room. We weren't sure what he was doing. David said, "Oh, ignore him. He can't get out." Fighting exhaustion, I got up and quietly opened our bedroom door to look. I was shocked. He was trying to remove the hinges on the door to the garage! I walked closer to see what kind of *tools* he was using: scissors, nail clippers, and a piece of wood.

These nighttime explorations were wearing us down. But our consciences prevented us from sleeping soundly. Ignoring Mardig was no way to treat a human being. We tried to rationalize our behavior. Ignoring him when he wasn't in any danger was the only way we knew how to cope. We weren't being good caregivers. *A parent would get up and comfort the child.*

"What do you mean?" David tried to delay answering my father's question.

"Someone has taken my shoes," Mardig clarified.

"We have them," I volunteered, trying an honest approach.

"Why?"

"Because we don't want you wearing them in the house," I said.

"Why did you take *my* shoes?" Mardig insisted.

"Because you wear them *in* the house," David answered firmly.

"Where are my shoes?"

"We have them," I said.

"They are *my* shoes," he emphasized.

"Yes, I know they are yours. And you will get them when you need to leave the house," I added.

"I'm leaving *now*!"

"At three in the morning?" David asked.

"That doesn't matter. I want *my* shoes."

The same evening, after dinner, Mardig surprised us. Looking genuinely perplexed, he spoke slowly, "You know, I take my shoes off and put them under the bed, and then they disappear. Do you know where they are?"

David and I shot glances at each other. Was he testing us?

"Yes, we have them," I said.

"*You* have them?" he asked, surprised.

"Yes," David said.

He chuckled, "Why do *you* need my shoes?"

We weren't sure if he was humoring us or if he truly was curious. *Was this Mardig talking in a lucid moment or the disease?*

Mornings and evenings, every single day, my father asked, "Where's my shoes?" David and I agreed we'd never be able to hear that question from anyone without having a reaction. Surprisingly, we found a benefit in hiding his shoes. Not having shoes created an obstacle to his leaving. With his shoes missing, Mardig's attention was first directed to finding them.

Eventually, Mardig came up with his own strategy. He began

hiding his shoes from us! First, he pushed them further underneath the bed. We found and removed them. Then, he hid them behind the rocker by the bookshelf. Next, he hid them behind some boxes in the closet; and then, behind the doors to one of the bookshelves. These last two hiding places really challenged us. We returned to his room repeatedly under the guise of seeing how he was doing or bidding him good night. While one of us searched, the other engaged him. Then he left his shoes in an obvious place, in the utility room where we keep ours. *Wait a minute. He tricked us. David's shoes are missing!*

With the Thanksgiving holiday approaching, David's parents invited us to their home in Las Vegas for a nice family dinner and maybe some gambling at the casinos. David's mother thought Mardig would enjoy the visit. *David's family also removes their shoes before walking in their home. We laughed at the thought of a new venue for shoe removal. If Mardig wasn't confused already, he might wonder why "every" place he goes requires him to remove his shoes.* We didn't know how Mardig would react, but we thought the adventure would be good. We packed an overnight bag for him with extras, and his moccasins, and started early Thanksgiving morning. I sat in the backseat with a video camera and Mardig sat in front with David.

The four-hour drive to Las Vegas was uneventful. David and Mardig talked. I napped and occasionally shot some footage, especially when we approached the Strip with all the new buildings, electronic billboards, and colors vying for our attention. Mardig was surprised we were in Las Vegas. I think he thought we made the four-hour trip by car from Wisconsin, not California.

We stopped at a grocery store near my in-laws' home to pick up some goodies. Once we arrived at their house, I stood back with the video camera, hoping to catch the moment the door opened and David's parents saw my father. I doubt Mardig remembered who we were visiting. Still it was such a joy to see David's mother greet my father with a big smile and a hug. None of us knew what to expect. It didn't take long, however, for all of us to settle in and feel at home while enjoying one another's company. *I neglected to notice if David or his family asked Mardig to remove his shoes.*

Mardig read, watched a little television with David's brother, Bruce, and enjoyed the hearty Thanksgiving meal, even though he couldn't make sense of our dinner conversation and laughter. After Bruce finished eating, he picked up the video camera and zoomed in close without us realizing. We laughed when he replayed the extreme close-ups of our mouths as we talked or chewed dessert and wider shots of us gesturing.

That night, Mardig slept in the guest room and we slept on the floor in the living room. Because he wandered, we needed to ensure he wouldn't get outside. We slept lightly. Mardig got up during the night and was confused. He wanted to use the bathroom and didn't know where it was. David helped him find the bathroom and then explained where he was. After David's cajoling, Mardig went back to bed.

The following afternoon, we went to Caesar's Palace. David's father taught Mardig how to play the slot machines. We watched as Mardig enjoyed himself amidst the noise and flashing lights. He even won a few quarters! We took him to an IMAX feature film about whales. The screen was so huge we felt we were actually *on* the whale watching ship. Mardig enjoyed it, even though the sensation of motion made him feel seasick. We then went to a pub, and he asked for fish and chips. We enjoyed beer with our burgers and fries. Afterward, David and I took him to a candy store. He enjoyed the variety and colorful sweets! Like little kids, we each filled our small bags with candy.

It was late afternoon and there was a long drive ahead of us. We hugged David's parents, said our good-byes, and started the drive home. Mardig seemed fine. After sunset, we stopped for gas and I used the rest room. Mardig became confused and wanted to go back. He insisted we were headed in the wrong direction. *He was so convincing, we questioned whether we had made a wrong turn.* Mardig wanted to go back to *Milwaukee*. We struggled to help him understand. Eventually, he cooperated, but remained unconvinced.

We hoped that once we arrived home, he would see his things and be comforted by familiar surroundings. But we were not so fortunate. Mardig thought we were tricking him by reproducing his room and things in this *new* place. He insisted he had to go home, people were expecting him, and he would visit this place later. It took us a couple hours to get him to change into his pajamas and go to bed. He didn't understand, but thankfully was too tired from the travel to insist any longer.

We learned from other caregivers there's usually one behavior that really *gnaws* on a caregiver's nerves. It's different for each of us.

Mardig used a flat wooden toothpick to remove food particles stuck between his teeth. If it weren't frayed when he'd finished, he'd *save* it. We found used toothpicks on his bathroom counter, on bookshelves, propped in the bindings of hardcover books, on the stereo, on the kitchen counter, behind the stereo, in the computer's floppy disk drive slot, and on the recliner. The last one painfully poked me when I unknowingly sat on it. *Still, we were able to tolerate his toothpicks.*

Even the chewed bubblegum he saved by sticking it to the nightstand or on the external hard drive was tolerable. He'd laughingly say, "There's no sugar in it! I can chew it to clean my teeth without the sugar ruining my teeth!"

None of these things annoyed us as much as that incessant question, "Where's my shoes?"

CHAPTER 8

Medical Evaluation and Drug Study

B ert returned my call from the Center for Aging Research and Evaluation (CARE) at the Granada Hills Community Hospital.[1] Roberta highly recommended CARE when I inquired about qualified doctors to evaluate my father's condition. Other families at the adult day care center also praised CARE's team of specialists. With an upcoming business trip, I wanted to make sure Mardig was not facing any immediate health problems before I departed. Bert scheduled the initial evaluation for the following week.

Up until now, Mardig had gone to the neighborhood clinic in Milwaukee for his health care. Although they did a fine job, my father did not always follow through with their suggestions. I would be actively involved, so I wanted him to be seen by dedicated specialists. Marlene Harrison, Director of CARE, called a few days later to ask questions as part of the pre-visit assessment. I felt a little uneasy answering medical questions on behalf of my father. It was difficult getting used to being responsible for another adult, one whose medical history was beginning to unfold. It started my affirmative response to twenty-two of twenty-nine listed functional/cognitive impairments.

---

1 The Granada Hills Community Hospital and Center of Research and Evaluation closed in 2003 having succumbed to financial difficulties.

After a one-hour drive to the San Fernando Valley (just north of Los Angeles), Mardig and I reviewed and signed the standard admissions paperwork. We found the CARE staff to be warm and thoughtful, even when Mardig asked questions that didn't make sense. Mardig was pleased with the attention he was receiving. The staff operated smoothly and easily interacted with him. I was confident Mardig would receive a thorough evaluation.

For the first two and a half hours they asked questions about his medical history, checked his vital signs (blood pressure, heart rate, body temperature, height, and weight), and more. They took blood and urine samples and asked him questions to evaluate his awareness and recall. Dr. Weinberg, a neurologist who specializes in dementia, then saw Mardig. This mild-mannered and soft-spoken doctor also suggested a few additional items to follow up on as part of Mardig's care: have a podiatrist examine the fungal infection on Mardig's toes and check his ingrown toenail; schedule an eye exam before the dementia progressed so far that Mardig could no longer discriminate among the quality of images, for example, "Which can you see better, this or that?"; and visit a dermatologist for the skin sores on his legs. He was frequently scratching them.

During two subsequent visits to CARE, Mardig received every test imaginable to me. Among these was an X-ray (a matter of procedure since he did not have a recent one on record), an electrocardiogram (EKG) to monitor his heart, and an electroencephalogram (EEG) to monitor his brainwaves. He had to lay very still with his eyes closed for the EEG. During the twenty-minute reading, he opened his eyes and the machine went crazy! Despite this glitch, the technician said the initial readings appeared normal.

Mardig enjoyed the special treatment. Each time we returned to CARE, he talked about how fortunate he was for all the trouble I was going through just for him.

During our third visit to CARE, I asked Marlene for the results of the evaluation. She declined to tell me until a comprehensive report was put together. CARE uses a team concept where a gerontological registered nurse, neurologist, psychologist, pharmacist, and other representatives meet to discuss each patient's case. Out of this meeting comes a comprehensive report. In this day of five-minute assembly line care; I was surprised to see so much time dedicated to my father.

When all was finished, I was given a twenty-page, mostly single-spaced, typed report; plus an in-person briefing. The report presented an elaborate background history, social and family history, results of the physical and neuropsychological examinations, and overall comments. I was impressed. They found a slightly elevated B.U.N. (blood urine nitrogen) and explained this may be due to Mardig not drinking enough liquids, which caused a bit of internal bleeding. They recommended testing his stool for occult blood. The EEG yielded no brain seizure activity. Mardig scored a nineteen out of thirty using the Folstein Mini Mental Status Exam. Diagnosis: "dementia, probable Alzheimer's."

Mardig also had a most informative verbal evaluation of his speech, language, cognition, and memory. Marlys Meckler went beyond the role of speech pathologist and gave us thirty-two suggestions to help us better care for him, among them:

◆ Label each door in the house to make it easier for my father to orient himself. Using the computer, we made huge labels with three-inch letters and taped them to each door: OUTSIDE, MARDIG'S ROOM, BRENDA'S OFFICE, DAVID & BRENDA'S BEDROOM, GARAGE DOOR.

◆ To get Mardig's attention, establish eye contact and gently touch him while speaking in a calming voice.

◆ Urge him to use his hearing aid. During the meeting, she showed us how to use it.

◆ Share photos of family members to better orient him. We created a photo album.

◆ Tell him on the day he's scheduled for an appointment, instead of earlier, so he doesn't get anxious.

◆ Break all activities, like dressing, into simple steps: "Put on your shirt." "Here are your pants." "Put on your jacket." "Remember your glasses."

◆ Get an identification bracelet for him or enroll him in the national Safe Return™ Program. Should he get lost, the authorities could easily identify him. We had already arranged this through the adult day care center.

My immediate concern was answered; there was nothing requiring immediate action.

Within one month after my business trip, Mardig had seen most of the doctors and specialists, including a dermatologist, audiologist, ophthalmologist, and dentist.

Each time I drove my father the fifty-two miles to CARE, I felt like his parent. I had taken him to more doctors than I had seen myself. I was making sure every detail of his health was evaluated and documented.

December 1996, only three months after Mardig moved to California, we were given the opportunity to enroll him in a drug study. Donepezil hydrochloride (Aricept®), had been approved by the U.S. Food and Drug Administration (FDA) in November for early to moderate Alzheimer's. Eisai America, Inc. (headquartered in Tokyo, Japan) was sponsoring the study to evaluate its safety and effectiveness. Preliminary findings showed it was beneficial in the treatment of people with Alzheimer's. All study participants would receive the actual drug in five- or ten-milligram doses.

This was the first time Alzheimer's, not just dementia, was mentioned with any regularity in reference to my father. David and I talked with Dr. Jacobs, who was conducting the study, and with Dr.

Weinberg, who initially examined Mardig. We asked many questions about Aricept® and read the small print provided to the U.S. by Eisai and Pfizer.

In order to be accepted into the study, Mardig had to pass an initial screening like the one he had in September. He would also be tested for syphilis since its symptoms occasionally are similar to Alzheimer's disease. If he passed these tests, we could return for his baseline exam, in order to document his current condition and start him on the medication.

We wanted Mardig in this study for two reasons. First, Aricept® might actually help him. He had been declining noticeably during the last few weeks and we wished he could improve enough to manage his own affairs. His financial affairs had taken far more time than we ever anticipated. *He may even be able to move back to his home!* This was our fantasy. Kim Wilms, the study coordinator, assured us no such improvement had been documented.

Second, the Aricept® study would place him under the intense scrutiny of a doctor for eight visits across forty-eight weeks. This was certainly an advantage, since the FDA's special requirements ensured quality of care. Besides, I knew my father would be supportive of a doctor-supervised study that might help him improve.

It was also during this time Dr. Weinberg finally put my father's condition in print: "dementia of the Alzheimer's type."

I asked more questions of Dr. Jacobs, an uncommonly attired doctor, because I wanted to be sure I was making the right decision on my father's behalf. It took me some time to get used to a doctor who donned cowboy gear—a loose denim shirt unbuttoned at the collar, tight-fitting jeans with a belt, and the requisite oversized buckle, finished off with cowboy boots. I later learned this personable and knowledgeable doctor rode to and from work on a motorcycle. *My father is about to embark on a clinical study with a motorcycle-riding cowboy!*

Mardig seemed unfazed by Dr. Jacobs' attire; he never said a word about it. We signed the study contract and I agreed to provide CARE with regular reports of Mardig's condition.

In mid-December I started keeping a daily journal for the study. I jotted notes whenever I could. What follows is most of the entire journal in its original and unedited form.

WEDNESDAY, DECEMBER 18, 1996

Took Mardig to CARE. A funny thing happened during Mardig's mental evaluation. Mardig was asked to name as many words as he could, beginning with "s." Mardig's first word was "sex." In contrast to his condition, the number of three syllable words he effortlessly listed proved that all those years spent reading had served him well. Accepted into drug study. Took first pill (5 mg.) at 5:10 p.m. while still at CARE.

Went to dinner in North Hollywood (to celebrate and to avoid traffic going home). After seeing the "Hollywood" street sign, Mardig could not believe "Hollywood" was in Chicago. He suggested spending the night in a hotel. After dinner, he didn't want to drive a long time. (He probably thought we were farther away than we were.) Arrived home at 10:00 p.m. . . . amazed at how all his stuff was here . . . how it looked the same. Wanted to leave . . . got mean . . . said unkind things.

THURSDAY, DECEMBER 19, 1996

8:00 a.m. Talked about his terrible dream last night. 9:00 appointment with attorney in order to determine his capacity to understand and sign estate-planning documents. Arrived at 9:30. Mardig still disoriented. Attorney asked questions, Mardig answered.

"Do you own your own home?"

"Yes."

"What city is it in?"

"Milwaukee."

"Do you remember the address?"

No answer.

"How much money do you think you have in the bank?"

"Seventy thousand dollars."

"Other than money in the bank, do you have any stock or bonds?"

"Those are included."

"Is your wife still living?"

"Yes, she lives in New York."

"Do you have any children?"

"Yes."

"How many?"

"Four."

Predictably, Mardig did not pass the test.

At 10:45 a.m. I took him to the adult day care center.

At night, he said he was going to bed. I gave him an Aricept® tablet with water. After he took it, he stayed up for another four hours.

FRIDAY, DECEMBER 20, 1996

Irritated . . . came into my office, twice within five minutes, asking where he can go for a haircut. Couldn't hear my answer. Wouldn't wear hearing aid. Wanted shoes.

SATURDAY, DECEMBER 21, 1996

Agitated. Incident where he wore shoes in the house and refused to take them off.

Went out in backyard . . . looked around for something? Came inside and then went out a second time and was gone! Jumped the fence! David took his cell phone and went on foot to find him. Followed him at a distance for 40 minutes . . . Mardig asked strangers where he lived . . . tried to evade David.

I came later with the car and picked up David. Driving alongside while Mardig was walking, we tried to persuade him to come into the car. He refused. We retreated awhile, tracking him from a comfortable distance. Then I started losing patience. Once he reached the busy street we decided to use force if necessary to get him in the car. We were afraid of him walking alone on a busy street. My adrenaline rushing, I stopped the car in the far right lane of the six-lane street. I turned on the hazard lights and left it running. As Mardig's POA, I told David to do whatever it took to get him in the car. I didn't want any battery charges because a son-in-law used physical force. *This was like kidnapping. We've seen it on television. A van screeches to a halt next to a playground. A person jumps out, snatches a child, and then jumps back into the van. The van then speeds away.* We were afraid, shaking, wondering what we would say if someone saw us and interfered. We had to act fast.

David and I got on each side of Mardig, and lifted him up from under his arms and carried him kicking and screaming a few yards to the car. I turned him around to face me and tried to push him into the backseat of the car. He wouldn't lower his head. Remembering something I'd seen on TV, I tried to get him to bend by applying pressure to his stomach. It worked; he bent and then screamed his head was hitting the car. My hand had been on top of his head with two inches to spare. Once we got him inside the car, I asked David to sit in the backseat with him. I drove with Mardig ranting and raving that kidnapping is against the law and he could have us arrested for hurting him. I told him we were doing this for his own good. I offered to take him to the sheriff's station so he could file a report if he really believed we did wrong. He continued complaining, so I drove to the station and asked him if he wanted to get out and file a report. He hesitated. I even volunteered to come inside with him. He refused to go inside. He said it would get us in trouble and he didn't want to hurt us. *Phew!*

After I pulled the car into the attached garage and closed the door, I had to cajole him back into the house. He was concerned about losing face if he came into house. David, who was shaken by this whole experience, had already gone inside. I tried to encourage my father. Later, and with a lot of prompting, he came in, ate some snacks, and then tried to play a game of backgammon. I knew things were starting to turn for the better, when he said, "My brain is too small to learn such a complex game!"

SUNDAY, DECEMBER 22, 1996

Some obstinateness and appearance of depression. Stayed in his room. We brought him his newspaper and warm chocolate milk. He came out later and helped us make breakfast by frying the bacon. We discussed finances after breakfast . . . he wanted to strategize how to keep his finances a secret . . . "Just you and me need to know," he said to me. Insisted on finding his wallet before we went shopping. We looked for 20 minutes. He forgot what he was looking for.

MONDAY, DECEMBER 23, 1996 (DAVID'S NOTES)

Irritated about the Safe Return™ bracelet. Kept trying to take it off. Always speaks of his shoes being taken. Seemed depressed in evening.

WEDNESDAY, DECEMBER 25, 1996 (DAVID'S NOTES)

Got up. Wanted his shoes in order to leave to do his job. Kept insisting he had to leave. Wanted to leave, wearing his pajamas. Was very irritated in the morning before we left. We drove a friend to the Burbank Airport and then went to Oxnard to walk on the beach along the ocean. He was pleasant the rest of the day. We opened gifts in the evening while Brenda and I took turns videotaping it. Afterward, we watched a videotape from Thanksgiving in Las Vegas, our day in Oxnard at the ocean, and all of us opening our gifts. He recognized himself on TV!

THURSDAY, DECEMBER 26, 1996 (DAVID'S NOTES)

He ate candy at 5:30 a.m. I found the bag in the middle of the living room floor. He was so charged, he wanted to leave right away and go to work. He kept trying to leave the house. I took him to the Adult Day Care Center at 8:15.

He didn't want dinner when we came home. He went to bed at 6:30 p.m.—wanted to be ready for tomorrow.

(BRENDA'S NOTES)

Woke up at 10:40 p.m. and wanted to know when we were to leave . . . disoriented as to time of day . . . thought it was daytime . . . lost shaver . . . hid it in box in closet . . . didn't believe he did this. Wanted to lock things up so "they don't take and use them."

FRIDAY, DECEMBER 27, 1996 (DAVID'S NOTES)

Easy to deal with in the morning. Went to dermatologist. Appeared nervous. Removed hearing aid before doctor walked in room. Said doctor should talk loudly so we can get our money's worth.

SATURDAY, DECEMBER 28, 1996 (DAVID'S NOTES)

Woke up when heard him trying to leave. First question in the morning, "Where's my shoes?" After we convinced him he wasn't going anywhere, he settled down. This convincing took 1 1/2 hours. We went for a three-mile walk in the afternoon. He was cooperative. It appears parts of his memory are coming back. When asked, he remembered he had three children, knew his home address in Milwaukee, knew [Brenda's sister's] address, and he mentioned these things without hesitation. He knew these things in his slightly irritated state. It could be he knew these things just because he was mentally alert for some reason (up and down days), or the drug might be working. He also had a severe case of "Sundowner's syndrome." He insisted he had to go home. We couldn't help him understand this was home. He finally gave in but was a bit depressed because he started to realize he was confused as to where he was. His cognitive abilities seem to be improving—he has figured out how to open the large garage door (by pushing the button along the side of the doorway). He also figured out how to get out of the backyard—we think he broke the latch on the gate. I may be reading into it. But these are the things that are different.

SUNDAY, DECEMBER 29, 1996 (DAVID'S NOTES)

Read Sunday paper.

MONDAY, DECEMBER 30, 1996

Very cooperative. Aricept® seems to be working. Had #3 tooth pulled (due to infection and nerve damage) at about 3:00 p.m. He was not aware this would happen until about 30 minutes before. He was very apprehensive about it and did not really like the whole situation. Afterward, he stopped bleeding and felt no pain. He is on penicillin 4 times a day. I have Tylenol® #3 in case he needs it, but he has felt nothing. Went to bed about 8:30.

TUESDAY, DECEMBER 31, 1996 (DAVID'S NOTES)

Very cooperative and pleasant. It appears his cognitive abilities are improving—he was very interested in reading a story in *Reader's Digest*—he could even tell a little what the story was about. He is more able to maintain the thread of the conversation. His appetite seems to be increasing.

Went to bed about 8:00 p.m. and woke up at 12:00 a.m., got dressed and wanted to leave to go to work—could not understand the time—was irritated because we would not give him his shoes. Wanted to eat. We prepared a snack for him and then we went to bed. He stayed up for a while.

WEDNESDAY, JANUARY 1, 1997

For the first time in a long time (nearly four months), Mardig was able to sit and focus on one thing for two-and-a-half hours. He watched the colorful floats in the Rose Bowl Parade on TV. He was mesmerized! Then we took him to Mount Wilson overlooking Pasadena. He seemed to handle the altitude (5,600 feet) quite well, including the three-and-a-half narrow staircases up to the 100-inch Mt. Wilson telescope. We walked for quite a bit, in what turned out to be a cold drizzly day and he fared well. He was initially afraid as we were driving up the winding mountain road . . . "Slow down!" he'd yell, a little irritated. "Keep your eye on the road!"

Afterward, he was happy we made the trip. "This was really worth it!" he said.

THURSDAY, JANUARY 2, 1997

Mardig's cognitive ability appears to have declined. On the way home from day care he asked, "Where's Ma?" He hadn't asked this in awhile. He seemed surprised and unaware of his mother and mine (his wife) not being alive. Mardig admitted he couldn't even picture their faces. I showed him their pictures when we got home. He asked if there was anyone else like me (siblings) here. He laughed when I explained they were in Milwaukee and we were in California. He didn't believe he was in California.

I gave him a book to read, *Ring Around the Moon,* by Lois Erisey Poole, a local author. He read a few pages then set it aside with the comment, "I will digest it later."

FRIDAY, JANUARY 3, 1997

"Where's my shoes?" Ahh . . . welcome to the mornings with Mardig . . . every morning . . . rare not to hear this question.

Evening . . . Mardig watched TV. He didn't listen to the content so much as to the *meta-content* (how the message was delivered, the speaker's nationality and persuasiveness). When I asked him about the content he said he missed the beginning so he won't bother with the rest . . . he'll wait until later to digest it. After closing his eyes awhile, he asked if this was the same speaker he was watching earlier. He watched TV like this. It was almost as if interpreting the content was too difficult and so he commented on what he could see and the inflections he could hear. One thing can be said for him, he watches and follows more TV than before.

TUESDAY, JANUARY 7, 1997

It appears Mardig is experiencing more peaks and valleys. He seemed more alert and aware for two days and the other two days he seemed disoriented and confused.

THURSDAY, JANUARY 16, 1997

Mardig caught the flu Monday . . . was difficult at the day care center . . . when he came home he had 102° temperature. Gave him Tylenol® to bring down fever. Called CARE to report per requirements for participation in drug study.

Mardig started having bouts of incontinence—urinated on the floor in front of the toilet, in his pants—five incidents thus far.

Took Mardig to our doctor with a 101.5° fever. Didn't want to take any chances. Doctor prescribed antibiotic for partially infected (greenish) mucous.

MONDAY, JANUARY 20, 1997 (DAVID'S NOTES)

Kept asking, "Where's the flashlight?" while holding one. When I told him he had one in his hand, he said "Yeah, but where's the flashlight?" Really confused.

TUESDAY, JANUARY 21, 1997

Mardig seems to have declined in his ability to tell time. Does not know day from night by looking at the clock. His focus has also declined. It may also be that we are unable to keep on top of all his needs. We ask him to do one thing, and he does another. "Put in your hearing aid." He says, "Okay," and goes to his room and gets a toothpick.

There's a song he hums . . . used to hum it when he felt good. Now he hums it in order to feel good or hold onto a memory. We wish we could buy a recording of it, but we're not sure of the name. One friend thought it was called, *Good Night Irene*. We were unable to find this at the local music store.

A bit ornery—turns off hearing aid and then expects to converse. Can't hear and asks, "Huh?"

(DAVID'S NOTES)

No longer concerned about taxes—I don't think he knows or understands what taxes are—just signed papers without reading—unusual for him.

THURSDAY, JANUARY 23, 1997

8:30 a.m. After growing frustrations, cleaning up after his incontinence, his refusal to listen, and getting just plain exhausted keeping on top of everything, I was unable to cope and shared my displeasure with Mardig regarding not wearing his shoes in the house, his lack of concern for us, and more.

"Let me be until I die," he replied equally flustered.

Stubborn. Won't wear hearing aid. ("If you care for me you'll talk louder.")

Took him to adult day care.

When I picked him up in the afternoon, he said he liked the warmth of the car, because he felt chilled during the day. Refused to get out of the car when we came home. Sat in car while it was parked in garage. When I came out into the garage five minutes later, he said he wanted to sleep in car. I tried to convince him to come in but he wouldn't. I went back inside and then came out again, five minutes later. This time he motioned with his hand for me to go away. I could hear him humming a different tune!

We're getting less patient in dealing with him . . . getting tired.

One of the requirements of the drug study was a series of follow-up visits to monitor Mardig's condition while on Aricept®. One of those appointments was scheduled during a week in February when David and I would be out of town. Kim volunteered to drive the fifty-two miles to see my father.

On March 12th, I brought Mardig to CARE for his last follow-up visit because he no longer qualified for the study. I scrawled the following notes on three pieces of paper.

WEDNESDAY, MARCH 12, 1997

Trip down . . . asked questions all the way . . . one after another . . . like a child . . . chattering . . . asking same question ("Are you going to a particular place?") within five minutes of saying "Okay," to my answer.

He is now sitting next to me in an office here at CARE . . . humming and talking loudly . . . then pleading jokingly, "I wanna go home." Now reading a magazine . . . occupied . . . quiet.

Into my realm of awareness enters the sound of a man's voice asking, "Who am I here to see?" A woman answers. He repeats her answer, "Dr. Jacobs?" Then I hear, "Oh, okay." All is quiet and then I hear the question again, "Who am I here to see?" This happens several times. Must be the disease.

Dr. Jacobs reviewed notes . . . he says my father has moderate Alzheimer's—in the middle stage of Alzheimer's.

He then gave Mardig a little test. He drew a circle and told him it was a clock. He asked Mardig to write in the numbers of the clock. My father drew four little hash marks. Each was spaced equidistant from the other—one at the 12, another at 3, and the other two at 6 and 9. *This was a good start. He's going to do just fine!* He paused for a moment and then wrote the number 1 at the 10:00 position and ended with 3 at the 11:30 position. He then wrote the number 12 at the 1:00 position and ended with the number 2 at the 2:30 position. *What could he possibly be thinking?* The doctor asked if there was anything more. Mardig wrote the number 6 at the 5:00 position and then the numbers 7 through 10 were squeezed in the space occupied from 6:30 to 8:30.

Amazing. I sat quietly as I usually did while he was being tested. My desire to help Mardig was tempered by how privileged I felt to be able to stay in the room during these evaluations.

After the doctor finished, Aris, a staff member, entered. She had the same green booklet with the *Mini-Mental Status Exam* used during Mardig's previous visits. She asked him the same questions she had asked before. Mardig's answers would be compared to his earlier ones.

"What is today's date?" she asked.

"I don't care."

"What is . . . year?"

"Nineteen fifty-seven."

"Can you tell me what season it is?"

"Approaching winter."

"What country are we in?"

"We're in Russia."

"What state?"

"Used to be Wisconsin," my father said, laughing nervously.

". . . city?"

"Used to be Milwaukee, when I was small."

"What building are we in?"

"It's a federal item."

"What floor are we on?"

"First floor."

Throughout this question and answer period, Mardig repeatedly stopped and asked Aris questions. When he did not know the answer to one of her questions, he'd explain why he didn't know. This ten-minute test stretched out to twenty minutes.

Next, she asked him to spell "world." He managed this easily. Then she asked him to spell "world" backward. This is what he said, "d l r o" and then after pausing for a moment, he added, "l d."

She asked him to do a few more things.

"Close your eyes, Mr. Avadian."

He looked directly at her and said, "Close your eyes."

She repeated the request.

He covered his eyes. He sat there, with his left hand covering his left eye and his right hand covering his right eye, until she told him he could open his eyes.

She asked him to write a sentence on a blank sheet of paper. The sentence could be anything that came to his mind.

He wrote, "This teacher's too critical." During his last visit, he had written, "I hope I'm giving the right answers." During an earlier visit, he had written, "I hope this does some good." On another visit, he wrote a paragraph about not understanding why he was being evaluated.

She asked him to copy two pentagons already printed on another page in the book. Previously, he would effortlessly reproduce the geometric designs. This time Mardig could not easily reproduce them.

I felt sad witnessing my father's declining ability. On December 18, when he came in for the initial screening for this drug study, he received a rating of 21. A perfect score is 30. One week later, during the baseline exam for the study, he scored 17. Four weeks later, 16. Eight weeks later, 19. On this occasion, he scored a 14.

We would realize later, Aricept® delayed his decline. We had such strong expectations Mardig would improve enough to live his dreams—the dreams he kept putting off—we failed to see Aricept® helped him remain level. Once he was no longer taking the medication, he became noticeably worse. I could have continued to buy Aricept®, but David and I discussed it and decided it would be better to accept what is. *My father has Alzheimer's and there is not yet a cure.* I'll enjoy whatever time remains with my father.

CHAPTER 9

Support Group:
We Need Help!

Despite our dedication and efforts, David and I had to face our limitations and ask for help. I asked Roberta and the adult day care center staff questions nearly every time I dropped off my father in the morning and picked him up in the afternoon. Each time they'd answer my question and then suggest I attend the weekly caregiver support group meeting.

"What if my father locks himself in the bathroom and scalds himself while taking a shower?"

Roberta stood firm one morning, "Brenda, I'm sorry, but I'm not going to answer any more of your questions. You really need to attend the caregiver support group. Caregivers like you are dealing with the same things. They can answer all of your questions better than we can. I really think you will benefit from these meetings, Brenda."

"But I don't have time! I'm busy!" I whined.

"Well, you'll need to make the time, because we won't answer any more of your questions!"

I returned home upset. If I didn't have so much work to do, I would have driven right back there and taken my father out of that adult day care center. *Why couldn't they simply answer my questions?* As the morning wore on, I contemplated how I could fit a one-and-a-half-hour meeting into my week.

I had never attended a *support* group and knew I would feel uncomfortable sitting in a circle talking about my struggles and listening to everybody whine about their problems. I imagined a therapy session or an Alcoholics Anonymous meeting. Besides, I was much too busy. Between trying to manage my father's affairs and balance his needs with my consulting assignments and our personal and professional development network television business, where would I find the time?

I'd been burning the candle at both ends since my August-September trip to Milwaukee. Feeling hopeless and physically rundown, I was losing focus on building my businesses. Unable to spend time on my profession, I increasingly experienced resentment toward Mardig and especially at all the details surrounding his affairs. I was in over my head. I needed help!

I gave in. I would wake up at four-thirty in the morning in order to build in the extra time I would lose by attending the support group.

Seated around a long table were men and women in their fifties and older. I was the youngest and felt out of place. Half of the participants were caring for their spouses, and the others were caring for their parents. I sat quietly and listened while they took turns sharing their experiences, asking questions, and getting answers from one another. The ideas were so helpful to me; I took a full page of notes!

Finally, it was my turn. I didn't know what to say. There was a lot I wanted to talk about. I opted to give a quick overview.

"Hello. I am Brenda Avadian and am thirty-seven years old. My husband and I adopted my eighty-six-year-old father and moved him out of his Wisconsin home of forty-five years into our California home."

Some support group members chuckled at the idea of *adopting* my father, while one caregiver asked, "How did you manage to *adopt* your father?"

I laughed, "No, there was no formal adoption. This is what we call it, because he's dependent on us like a child."

"Do you have any sisters or brothers?"

"Yes, my forty-five-year-old brother still lives at home. He has not yet moved out of our parents' home. And my sister lives five blocks away."

"GASP! And they didn't help their father?"

"No, not really. The Milwaukee County Department of Aging called to let me know something was wrong."

I wanted their sympathy.

A soft-spoken woman hesitatingly asked, "Is your mother still living?"

I looked around to see who asked the question. Being deaf in my left ear, I could not tell where the sound was coming from.

She raised her hand and pointed toward herself.

"No, she died of congestive heart failure in 1993.

"Awww," I heard their collective voice of sadness.

Wow, this really felt good. These people understood what we were going through. They empathized and had good ideas!

Just then, the facilitator apologized and said we were out of time. *We were? We had an hour-and-a-half! The time went by too fast.* They invited me to return. Everyone began shuffling to leave.

"Bu-but, I have questions!" I blurted out. *I needed answers.*

"Oh, uh, all right. Since this is your first time . . . can everyone stay just a few more minutes?"

"Yes, yeah, sure," came the replies, as they laid their things on the table and sat back down.

"My father has difficulty getting his legs in and out of my car. What can I do to make it easier for him?"

"How big is your father?"

"A little over five feet."

"What kind of car do you drive?"

"A Mazda Miata convertible."

"Get a new car!" they laughed.

Smiling at their humor, I said, "That's not an option right now. Besides I like my small car!"

One of the women spoke up. "My husband's a big man and his legs get very stiff. I folded a heavy-duty plastic garbage bag in half on the seat. He can easily pivot around on the slippery bag to get in and out of the car."

"That's a *great* idea!" I exclaimed, quickly jotting down a note. "Okay, I have one more question. What if my father locks himself in the bathroom and scalds himself while taking a shower?"

"Yeah, that's a good question," one of the men replied. "I keep an ice pick handy to put in the little hole to unlock the door from the outside."

"An ice pick?" I asked, wondering if the bathroom doorknob even had a little hole.

Another caregiver added, "Or a jeweler's screwdriver."

"A jeweler's screwdriver?"

"Yeah, those little screwdrivers you use to tighten your glasses. They are small enough to fit into the hole."

I jotted more notes down and thanked them for their help.

The meeting was over. I gathered my things and walked out of the meeting room to the bigger room where the participants were engaged in activities as they waited for their family members to pick them up. My father was seated next to another participant at the table. He had a pile of magazines with lots of pictures in front of him.

"Mardig, your workday is finished. You can come home now," I told him.

He looked inquisitively at one of the activity aides for confirmation.

She nodded, "Thank you for all your help, Marty. We really appreciate it! Hope we'll see you tomorrow!"

He smiled, "You will. I'll come bright 'n early!"

"Not too early," she jested. "We might not be open yet!"

Once we got home, I handed him the keys so he could walk to the middle of the block and get our mail from the bank of mailboxes. When he returned with our mail, we walked inside. On the way to the family room, I looked at the bathroom doorknob. Luckily, it had a hole on the mounting plate. I grabbed a tiny screwdriver and played with the mechanism. After a few tries, it worked!

I attended meetings regularly after this. During the days between each support group meeting, I jotted down questions about caring for Mardig.

One day, a caregiver asked if it was normal for her mother to follow her instead of walking by her side. I smiled; I had the same question.

A few months after moving Mardig to California, we noticed when David and I went out with him he'd follow a few steps behind us. Or if I took him shopping, he'd say, "You go ahead. I'm coming." If I slowed down, he'd slow down, as if an invisible barrier was keeping us apart.

David and I thought this was strange. It was like a puppy was trailing behind. Sometimes, he was having a temper tantrum and wanted to keep his distance.

The support group offered another explanation: People with Alzheimer's follow because they feel safer being able to see their caregivers in front of them.

Whatever the reason, it posed a problem for us when Mardig was distracted and walked somewhere else. We had to retrace our steps to find him.

Each caregiver was at a different stage of the caregiving experience, so the meetings were helpful.

"You are now the parent and need to be firm with your loved one for his own safety."

"Get satin sheets so your loved one can slide in and out of bed easier." *Oops! We had just ordered thick flannel sheets so Mardig would be comfortable and warm.*

"You will be glad you took on this responsibility in the end."

Yes, if I live that long and don't lose my income! My consulting practice of seventeen years was slowly slipping from my hands and our television network business suffered from neglect as my focus turned toward caring for my father.

The upside was all the information shared during the support group meetings. Some of us formed a bond that ultimately carried me through years of highs and lows. The support group became my second family. We had something in common: one of our family members had dementia or Alzheimer's. No one can completely understand what it's like caring for someone with Alzheimer's unless he or she is a caregiver.

Patti, only in her early fifties, cared for her sixty-two-year-old husband. He had the bluest eyes and the most striking wavy white hair.

Paul, who was in his early eighties, consistently shared at least one profound nugget at each meeting, that made us think. He was progressive enough to have an Internet account and was adding features I had not even considered; for example, voice recognition software and a digital camera.

Jonathan, at eighty-three, cared for his wife, and like Paul, also had an Internet account.

Paul and Jonathan had been married to their wives for more than fifty years before symptoms of Alzheimer's took over. Patti enjoyed ten years with Ralph before he yielded to the clutches of Alzheimer's.

Jeanne, a nurse, gave up her career to care for her mother in her own home. She was in her early fifties.

Other caregivers attended these meetings, but Patti, Paul, Jonathan, and Jeanne attended consistently and were of the most help to me.

Throughout the highs and the lows, I missed having a supportive relationship with my sister and brother. *Didn't they care? Why weren't they calling?* To survive, I was creating my own family of friends.

The support group and the book, *The 36-Hour Day*, by Nancy L. Mace and Peter V. Rabins, became two key items in my caregiver survival kit. I dubbed this book, "The Caregiver's Bible." The cover reads, "A family guide to caring for persons with Alzheimer's disease, related dementing illness, and memory loss in later life." Each caregiver who wanted to survive the experience had a copy. When something happened, we'd refer to the appropriate section in the book for help. Sometimes the answers were painfully graphic; other times, they weren't specific enough.

But the support group was there, week after week, to fill in gaps of knowledge and extend support, especially during the hopeless times.

During a particularly trying week in October 1996, I recorded the following in my journal.

OCTOBER 1996

Last night was awful . . . I was very sick. The flu hit me severely, and Mardig was not being cooperative. He went to bed around 10:00 p.m. and so did I. I was having terrible chills. The quartz heater was turned on high to warm me under three covers and I still could not combat the chills. David was cleaning up the kitchen after he made chicken soup for us.

David came to bed about 10:30. Mardig was in his room and the lights were turned off. At 11:00, we noticed the lights go on. Hell was about to begin . . .

Mardig got out of his room; all dressed, and was ready to leave. He started wandering around in the house wearing his shoes. He was opening doors, cupboards, including the front door eight times (it makes a scraping noise so we knew). I didn't want to get up because I was freezing. Mardig quietly went into the utility room, turned on the lights, and then turned them off. We couldn't make sense of what we were not hearing. He must have just stood there in the dark. David got up and peered down the hallway from our bedroom door. Who knows what my father was doing. I feared he might hurt himself. (I think we need to childproof this house so he doesn't get hurt.)

After that, David got up six or seven times. It was 3:00 a.m. and David had to get up in an hour to leave by 4:55 a.m. He was too exhausted. He just couldn't take it anymore. I got up at 3:30 a.m. and looked around.

David's files of his parents' tax and business records had been opened. The organized piles on my desk had been mixed up. Each pile was for a different project. It took me time to organize my work. During the few hours I had each day to work, I certainly didn't have time to reorganize after someone else messed my files! I was cold, very cold. I lost patience. What happens if I get hurt or truly can't get up? How will I take care of my father? This was inappropriate . . . Mardig was causing too much trouble. Battling severe chills, I had enough . . . I confronted Mardig and told him this couldn't go on any longer. He told me to leave him alone. I said I couldn't because he was messing up my stuff and affecting my life! He told me to leave him be, he would die soon. *Ooooohhh, he used the ultimate guilt-rendering tactic!*

The following morning, I found a small block of bittersweet baking chocolate on the floor by the kitchen sink. *We keep it in the cupboards high above Mardig's head.* I found a spoon in the toaster. *It's a good thing we always unplug the toaster.* When I told Mardig about this he was amazed and denied he'd do anything so stupid—"You could get a shock!" he added. I found the jar of peanut butter among the cleaning supplies under the sink.

That afternoon, he pulled out a slice of bread from the bag, after I had already given him one to have with his soda. (He liked to eat bread and wash it down with sweet creamy soda.) When I came into the kitchen, both pieces of bread were placed on one of the cat's food bowls at the edge of the counter. I made him aware of what he had done. He thanked me for looking out for him. I threw the bread out for the birds and retrieved another couple of slices for him. I have to constantly keep an eye on him so he doesn't harm himself.

We will have to try sleeping pills for Mardig. We'll see how they help him sleep. It'll be good for him and us. Other caregivers at the support group recommended this. The first night the sleeping pills worked. The next two nights he was up wandering, so we stopped giving him sleeping pills after the third night.

I started researching our options for assisted care for him. We'll check one out this weekend. It is just too difficult to constantly watch him each time he gets up.

I feel the dual emotions of sadness and relief . . . David says Mardig is eighty-six. He's lived his life, now we must live ours. I agree. On the other hand, Mardig seems so helpless, so innocent. His being here has taught me much about options. Life is full of them! And it's not like he's doing this on purpose. Yeah, sometimes he's ornery just to be stubborn, but most of the time, he doesn't realize he's being bothersome.

After incidents like these and while I was feeling particularly weak and helpless, I brought up the question I hesitated to ask the support group, because it would mean I had failed. "How do you know when you can't do it anymore? When you just can't care for your loved one."

"You'll know," one said. "We can't tell you, because it's different for everyone," Paul added.

How disappointing! What an easy way not to answer the question. This is not what I needed, especially from my support group family! I had never taken care of someone with dementia before. How will I know when I can't do it anymore?

They were right! During those months, I learned *how right* they were. Each of us has our limits. We wanted to give up many times. "Let's just take him back to Milwaukee and leave him there! We don't owe him anything! We've already given him more than anyone else in the family has."

But we couldn't take Mardig back. We had taken on this responsibility. We had to see it through. David and I made sacrifices. Weekends and evenings were devoted to my father's care. Our relationship was sorely neglected. Our focus was entirely on our eighty-six-year-old child. We planned meals around his nutritional needs, doctors' visits were arranged for him, and fun outings were planned just for him.

Having lived together for nineteen years, David and I no longer enjoyed dinners out as a couple or spent time with friends. We couldn't even enjoy our outdoor Jacuzzi because we feared what Mardig might do inside the house. With my attention focused on Mardig's whereabouts, I couldn't feel relaxed with David in bed. My attention was fixed outside our bedroom door.

And, despite everything we were doing for Mardig, he was still declining. Were we doing something wrong? Were we not doing enough?

One day after I dropped him off at the adult day care center, I asked several staff members about this. One staff member painted a vivid picture for me. She said, "Your father is like a drunk who's trying to hold it all together in public. If someone asks him a question, he will answer intelligently. This takes a lot of effort. But once he gets in a private place where he feels safe, like your home, he relaxes. And this means he may not make sense."

It took me a while to understand her example and to accept this analogy. *By doing good things for Mardig and making him feel safe, he was able to feel comfortable enough to relax. This allowed the disease to progress along its natural course.*

Still, I was exhausted! Mardig's erratic sleep schedule, increased disorientation and confusion, fever, and bouts of incontinence were taking their toll. Mardig refused to stay away from me while I had the flu. He'd touch my hand and then eat without washing his hands first. "What's a little germ?" he'd tease, when David and I urged him to wash his hands. I stayed home each day and parented my father who had caught the flu from me.

He became disoriented and suffered two major rounds of incontinence. He didn't know the time of day and was not making sense. I was concerned about keeping his fever down. I called the doctor in a panic when his fever rose to 103° with no signs of abating. The doctor advised trying Tylenol® (acetaminophen). It worked quickly. Every few hours when his temperature started creeping back up I'd take his temperature and give him Tylenol®.

I discovered the depths of my compassion for Mardig during this time. Fecal matter fell out of his pant leg as I led him to the bathroom. I helped him onto the toilet and then went back to clean up the mess. *Yuck! I stepped on feces in his bedroom!*

Mardig ate the dry cat food stored in a sealed plastic container on the kitchen counter. He became so constipated he had a bowel movement whenever and wherever he could. Then he had diarrhea. We found feces in his bedroom, in the hallway, and in the living room. *We definitely needed to have the carpets cleaned.*

I would wake at 4:30 each morning with the goal of getting some work done. First, I'd check his bathroom. "It was easier to clean a small mess than a big one," I reasoned. I found feces and urine on the floor and his soiled underwear in the sink. *If his underwear was in the sink, what was he (not) wearing?* I began each morning with a bottle of bleach, plenty of paper towels, and wiped his bathroom clean. What a way to start each day.

Without the support group I would have felt alone, misunderstood, and lost. I would not have been able to survive the trying times. As caregivers openly shared their most personal experiences, I was better able to understand what Mardig was going through and what to expect. Their experiences opened my eyes and caring for my father was filled with fewer surprises. With their support, especially through those particularly treacherous days of twenty-four-hour-a-day care, I learned and gained enough confidence as a caregiver, to start sharing my ideas and experiences with others.

We were truly a *support* group because we encouraged one another and drew on one another's strengths as we provided quality care for our loved ones. Our trust, mutual respect, and emotional bonds deepened as we grew into a *family*. We helped one another, got together during the holidays, and had a wonderful time knowing support was a short distance away. I'm glad I made time to become a member of my support group family . . . for my father's sake and mine!

CHAPTER 10

Money, Money, Money

"How much do I have?" While in Milwaukee in March 1996, my father invited me to go with him to the bank. He said he needed to take care of a few things. His bank was a half-mile away, and he wanted to walk for exercise. I said I'd accompany him. It would be a good opportunity for us to be outdoors on a mild winter day. At nearly fifty years his junior, I could barely keep up with his rapid stride, much less carry on a conversation without getting out of breath.

At the bank, I felt funny standing near him while he did his banking. I tried to appear uninterested and began thinking about my teenage years. My parents had kept their financial affairs private. When I applied for a financial aid grant to attend the University of Wisconsin-Milwaukee, they refused to complete the paperwork. They didn't want anyone to know about their finances.

My thoughts were interrupted by the customer service representative's curt voice, "Mr. Avadian, you came here two days ago asking for that information."

"Well, *now* I want it," Mardig said with emphasis.

"We gave you a printout of what you have!"

I wondered if she was being unnecessarily rude, so I began to pay attention. I stepped closer to Mardig and asked him what he needed. He looked at me briefly and then looked back at the woman and demanded, "I want to know what I have in my accounts."

Flustered, she relented, "Okay, I'll give you another printout."

Having succeeded, he looked at me with glee. I asked him what he was trying to do. He explained he didn't want the bank to forget about his money so he had to keep track of what he owned.

Mardig then shifted his focus to some brochures. I used his distraction to introduce myself to the representative as she waited for the account information to finish printing.

She apologized for her behavior and said Mardig came to the bank three times a week asking about his money.

I was surprised. I couldn't believe he was so preoccupied with his accounts. "Really?" I asked.

"Yes," she said moving her gaze downward toward her desk.

"Why?"

"He forgets," she said.

"Wow, that must get kind of irritating," I added.

She looked up with a smile and asked in seeming disbelief, "You're his daughter?"

"Yes, I am." I stood a little taller, having introduced myself earlier.

"Well, you should have him give you power of attorney so you can help him with his finances."

"What?"

"Yes, with a POA you can help him keep track of his accounts so he doesn't have to worry as much." *Since I never quite measured up to my older brother or sister—in their and sometimes even in my parents' eyes—my heart raced with excitement. Did she really invite me to get involved with my father's money?* I calmed myself and said, "I'll think about it. My father has two other children who should be involved."

I walked away feeling a sense of vindication. I had been invited to enter the secret domain of my father's finances. WOW, I was tickled!

∽∽

Days later, Mardig asked me to help him with his finances. "Talk with the bank and I will coach you to make sure they don't cheat us."

"Which bank?" I asked. When he told me, I replied with surprise, "But we just went to that bank, Mardig!"

"I don't want them to cheat us. Let's go *now!*" He glanced at David, who was standing in the kitchen with us and then looked back at me, "Hey, he can come with us. We need witnesses."

Mardig stood next to me with pride as I became his right arm and got what he wanted from the bank. It was then he gave me POA.

Happy with his success, he said, "Let's go to the other bank. Now I want you to ask for . . ."

All this was moving too fast. From hardly knowing anything about his finances, I was getting more involved. I was afraid. I repeatedly asked my sister and brother to be involved in Mardig's care and affairs, they didn't respond. I felt alone. I didn't want to be perceived as the child who flew into town for Mardig's money.

Despite this ambivalence, when David and I watched a repeat performance at Mardig's second bank, David suggested to Mardig that he give me POA. Mardig declined. I thought, It's his business.

Five months later, in August, Mardig and I returned to his first bank. Even after he gave me POA of this account, my words were being ignored. "Mardig, that's not a check. It's a *copy* of a check."

"Shhh," he said sternly, and then demanded the teller cash the check.

"Mr. Avadian, we can't accept this. It is not a negotiable document."

"What do you mean, you can't accept this? Look, it's a check!"

"Mardig," I retrieved the check, "this is a *copy* of a check, see?" I showed him both sides of the full-sized sheet of paper onto which the check had been copied. "Besides, look, there's even a copy of your signature here on the back. You must have cashed it earlier."

Mardig walked away. I smiled sheepishly at the teller and followed Mardig to the representative we met in March.

"May I have a copy of my account information?" he asked politely.

I stood by helpless. The representative gave me an empathic smile; I reciprocated. *We both felt helpless when faced with Mardig's conviction.*

With copies in hand, we left the bank and Mardig said, "Let's check on the others."

"The others?"

I watched as he headed in the opposite direction from where we parked the car. I caught up to him and we walked a couple blocks to his other bank. He walked over to a friendly bank representative who invited us to sit down. The young man and Mardig conversed easily and smiled a lot. Mardig didn't want to renew a certificate of deposit. He feared he would forget to cancel the renewal. He asked if I could follow up to make sure the funds were transferred into his savings account.

Mardig often told me he liked that I was keeping track of his papers. He was happy I could immediately answer his questions and show him proof of what he had. I really wasn't doing anything. As soon as I came across something, I'd show it to him, and I'd remember more of the details than he did. If I didn't remember, I'd find the paperwork, if he hadn't misplaced it.

The representative explained to him he'd need to give me power of attorney or add my name to the account, if Mardig wanted me to give direction to the bank regarding his account. My father agreed to give me power of attorney.

I felt dual emotions of happiness and worry. Hesitating, I asked, "Are you sure? What about [my sister] or [my brother]?" I felt awkward being involved with his finances and wanted to be fair. Besides, I didn't know what to expect from them.

Mardig said he didn't think my sister or brother should be involved. He gave me reasons that surprised me, yet strengthened my willingness to help him.

When David and I agreed to care for Mardig and handle his affairs, we were aware he owned General Electric stock and U.S. Savings Bonds. We knew he had two bank accounts. At best, we estimated his assets at $200,000.

This would be easy. Mardig had given me power of attorney. All I would have to do is transfer his accounts to California. The sooner we took care of these affairs; the sooner we could return to *normal* and his day-to-day care.

Once in California, we needed to open a bank account for Mardig. He said, "Since you're my attorney, you take care of it."

I laughed, "Nope, you need to come with me." We went to a neighborhood bank to establish an account in his name. While waiting for the representative to finish helping another couple, Mardig whispered, "You do the talking."

When she was finished, we approached her desk and sat down. "I'd like to open up a bank account for my father."

"Does he have identification?"

"Well, actually no. He seems to have misplaced his wallet." I leaned forward and said in a hushed voice, "He may have Alzheimer's." I sat up, then added, "However, I do have his POA, and I carry identification."

Appearing unaffected by my Alzheimer's comment, she replied, "We cannot open an account for him unless he has identification."

"Well, what do you need?"

"A driver's license or something with a photo ID and his signature."

"He no longer drives."

"Well, *you* could open an account."

"No, I don't want to open an account. I want this to be in his name with me as his POA." *My siblings' potential reactions to my name being on my father's account were reasons enough to keep things separate.*

She turned us down. Undeterred, we went to another bank. They would not let him open an account either. We tried one more bank. We were rejected. Mardig grew frustrated. I gave up. There was no sense in wasting time visiting each bank. *If these California banks didn't want my father's money, so be it.* We returned home and I decided to call the banks instead. "Hello, this is Brenda Avadian. I've lived here for seven years, shopped at the same neighborhood store, and banked at . . . can you help me?"

"No."

Not a single bank wanted Mardig's money, not without proper identification. And I didn't want to open an account for Mardig at our bank, because of the appearance to my siblings, of potentially co-mingling funds.

We applied for a credit card at one of Mardig's banks in Milwaukee. At least we could use it to pay his medical bills, buy him clothes, pay for gas after lengthy trips to the doctor, etc. We were unable to use his credit card as a form of identification, though.

These rejections initiated a long and frustrating chase around government bureaucracy including the Social Security Administration for his social security number and the Department of Motor Vehicles (DMV) for a California ID. It took one and a half months going from one government agency to the next and back again. It involved filling out paperwork, sitting in rooms filled with frustrated people listening for the next number to be called, waiting in line and once at the window being told to stand in the *correct line*, waiting again, being looked down upon, and being treated with suspicion. With only a shred of dignity remaining, Mardig and I emerged from the nightmarish bureaucratic maze with appropriate identification.

David and I discovered Mardig's savings bonds had expired. Thirty-nine of his thirty-plus-year-old savings bonds were no longer earning interest. Since we had not yet opened a bank account for him in California, I called the bank representative I had met in Milwaukee to arrange to cash the bonds.

David entered the bonds' serial numbers in the computer and Mardig signed each bond. *In California, he would have had to sign each in front of a notary. At $5 to $10 per signature, the fees would add up quickly!* We made a copy of the bonds for our records, in case they were lost, and then mailed them to the bank. We offered to keep the proceeds in his Milwaukee bank for several months. *Banks use deposits to provide loans at higher interest rates. We would be paying them back for helping us.* Besides, where else could we put the money?

One after the other, these little things added up. This constant running around kept us drowning in Mardig's affairs. We spent little time focused on anything else, let alone each other.

We needed an attorney who practiced law in the State of California. Attorney David Cohn had been helpful and I wanted to continue working with him; however, each state's laws are slightly different and it was necessary, with Mardig now in California, for us to proceed according to California law. David sent me a list of elder law attorneys who were members of the National Academy of Elder Law Attorneys (NAELA). Using this list and a trusted friend's recommendation, I met with a well-regarded attorney to discuss the best way to handle my father's affairs given a potentially contentious relationship with my siblings. After a fifteen-minute meeting, he advised that I do a conservatorship. He estimated the cost to be $5,500. *This is too much money! Plus, he made this decision too quickly!* I left his office with the impression he was trying to make easy money off me. I wanted more options. There had to be another way.

Trying to conserve expenses, I considered using paralegal services. After talking with two paralegals, I realized our situation demanded a custom approach.

The road ahead would be filled with costly potholes and more attorneys.

A referral from the support group to another elder law attorney put me face-to-face with one who was unlike any other attorney I had met. Her initial consultation lasted over an hour. She was more concerned, given my sibling situation, that a certified elder law attorney represent me. (She had not yet attained certification.) After giving away potential business, she even refused to charge me her fee! *This good deed would not be forgotten.*

We retained a certified elder law attorney practicing in California. His name was on the NAELA list and he came recommended. He helped us lay the groundwork for managing my father's affairs. With his connections, we opened a bank account in Mardig's name using the little identification we had for Mardig at the time. He also referred us to a certified public accountant who we retained to maintain records and provide an accounting of Mardig's finances. Every quarter, we'd gather Mardig's statements and check register, and take them to the accountant, so his staff could update Mardig's general ledger. We quickly learned the importance of creating an organized filing system to easily retrieve Mardig's records. We also documented everything.

I knew my sister and brother would not have had the patience to handle all these details. In fact, they would not have even discovered the details. My brother said, "I'll just dump everything. I have no time for all this junk, Brenda. I've got a business to run." This *junk* would include our father's U.S. Savings Bonds, information about his accounts across the country, and more. All told, this junk would be worth several times what we initially estimated.

My aunt and uncle had warned me that whenever families deal with money, strange things happen. "People do unreasonable things." So I kept accurate records and received the best guidance money could buy. I wanted to defend my actions confidently. If I had to stand in court, I wanted to face the judge squarely and speak unhesitatingly.

As the months passed, I became even more concerned about the uncertainty of my sister and brother's potential actions. Bitterness caused by the burden of managing Mardig's finances, hung like a heavy cloud over David and me. Caring for Mardig and managing his affairs involved an extraordinary commitment of time and thought. It was taking a heavy toll on David's and my businesses. I expressed these concerns each time I talked with the attorney. He suggested that a conservatorship would provide us with direction and approval from the court; thus, giving me the greater level of certainty I needed. I hesitated, given the cost and added time of organizing records for court approval. Besides, I walked out on this quick-fix approach earlier. I called Attorney Cohn and explained the situation and he still didn't think a conservatorship was necessary. He suggested we consider a revised power of attorney, incorporating the nuances of California law.

The legal details were beyond my understanding; I requested a teleconference among the three of us. I prepared thoroughly to maximize the time. *Imagine paying for two attorneys' time, simultaneously.* The outcome was the same. Our California attorney suggested petitioning the court for conservatorship. Mardig's Milwaukee attorney stayed with his initial suggestion of a revised POA.

I spent hours writing page after page of exactly what I was concerned about and why. I wanted compensation for my time since the estate was far more involved than initially expected and since it was taking time away from my professional work. If my sister and brother would share the responsibility, I'd feel differently. David and I had taken on this responsibility expecting only to care for Mardig and to handle a few simple financial details. Nothing prepared us for all the added responsibilities constantly hanging over our heads.

There was a large sum of money my brother had acquired through questionable means that still needed to be addressed. I wanted to ignore it, but there was the distinct possibility, years later, my sister could take me to court on the grounds I did not exercise my fiduciary responsibility to collect what's due. And how would I collect this money? Should I insist my brother return what he owed plus interest to the estate or should I consider annual cash gifts to my sister, her husband, my husband, and me? These gifts would help reduce the taxable size of the estate and move toward equalizing the benefit among us three siblings. These were options the attorneys had suggested. But what if we gave annual cash gifts and there wasn't enough left for my father's care? Questions like these kept swirling in my mind keeping me awake at night.

The California attorney agreed to redo the power of attorney according to California law and in consideration of my concerns. First, Mardig would have to prove he had the capacity to understand what he was signing. I set an appointment.

Mardig had a bad dream the night before we went to the attorney's office, so he was disoriented. I decided to take him anyway. The attorney asked a series of questions and Mardig was unable to answer them to the attorney's satisfaction. I decided not to wait for a moment of lucidity to pursue this POA. We would have to follow another course of action.

Three months before Mardig moved to California he believed his car had been stolen. "I'm not sure," he said between awkward chuckles, "but I think someone stole my car."

"Really?"

"Yeah . . . I drove the car up north and when it was dark I came home by bus."

"Up north?"

"Yeah, up north. You know where."

No, I didn't.

"I was afraid it was too dark and I'd get lost," he added with another chuckle. "So I parked the car somewhere and took the bus. I went to go find it in the morning and it was gone. Now they want money to get it back."

"Who wants money?"

"I dunno."

"Well, how much do they want to get it back?'

"A lot!"

"How much?"

"I dunno, maybe three or four hundred."

"Are you going to go get it?

"Naw," he said laughing. "That's too much money!"

The car was worth several thousand dollars.

David and I concluded he had illegally parked, so the city had it towed to a garage to be claimed. I asked my sister and brother about this; both agreed it was better our father did not have a car.

After Mardig moved in with us, he received a letter from a security supervisor at West Allis Memorial Hospital on Milwaukee's westside. (We had filed a "Change of Address" form with the post office so Mardig's mail would be forwarded to California.) The car had been abandoned for several months in their parking lot. The supervisor had used the license plate numbers to get the owner's information. *Did Mardig park it there and forget he drove somewhere? My sister mentioned he had done this before: drove somewhere, forgot, and ridden a bus home.* I called the security supervisor and explained the situation.

"Do you want to sell it?" he asked. "I'd like to buy it. I need a car and it looks like a nice car."

"Yes . . . Yes, I should talk with my sister first. She and her husband have only one car. Another car would make things a lot easier for them."

I tried to be considerate of my sister. Someday she'll appreciate my good intentions.

I called and started to leave a message offering her the car, when she picked up the phone. She sounded pleasant and we talked enthusiastically. We exchanged e-mails over the course of the next several weeks and worked through the details of transferring title from our father to her name. She said it would have been a lot easier if our brother let her into *his* house to look for the title to Mardig's car. *Then again, where would she find it?* In the end she was able to benefit from the last car our father drove.

Before the end of the year, both Attorney Cohn and our California attorney reviewed Mardig's accounting. After weighing how much the estate had grown compared to Mardig's modest expenses, we agreed a cash gift to my sister and me and to our hus-bands would reduce the estate tax burden without adversely affecting his future care needs. I couldn't wait to hear from my sister. She would be pleasantly surprised! The attorneys advised we subtract the fair market value of the car from my sister's portion of the gift. Surprisingly, I heard from my sister. She was angry with me. "I don't want the car if this is the result! I would never pay $2,300 for that car!" I shared her reaction with the attorneys; they didn't know what to say. *This is a first, attorneys with nothing to say!*

Another time-consuming detail that remained was, who really owned Mardig's house? My father frequently shared his fear that my brother owned the house and he needed to be careful around him so he wouldn't be left homeless. We weren't sure whose house it was. My brother claimed the house was his. We found undated and unsigned copies of a contract with my brother's name on it. I sent copies of these to Attorney David Cohn, and he offered to do a title search on the house. We waited for the results.

If the house were my brother's, it would save us a lot of work clearing out so many years' worth of my parents' belongings. We could just leave every-thing there. If, on the other hand, it were Mardig's, I would have to clear it out. How long would it take? Could others do this for me? Would they be as meticulous as I? Would someone help me? When would I find the time? I've already lost thousands of dollars worth of business because of all this work.

While we waited, Mardig's bills continued coming to our house. These included utility and property tax bills. If the house belonged to my brother, why was Mardig's name still on these bills? And why were some of the bills marked "overdue"?

We waited with anticipation while processing Mardig's extensive paperwork. *If the house were Mardig's, how would I get my brother to leave after living there his entire life?* David and I hoped my brother owned it. This would save us a lot of trouble.

As with most of life's worthy endeavors, our work was not easy—it was a *nightmare*. Mardig owned the house. My brother would have to move out so I could get it ready to sell. Evicting him would not be easy. I imagined telling him, "Dear brother, you've lived in this house for forty-five years for free. Don't you think it's time you moved out?"

There were laws to be followed, even when evicting a non-paying boarder. Mardig's attorney advised me and I composed a letter to my sister and brother that we had to clear out our father's home and our brother had to move so we could sell it. I invited them to help dispose of our parents' personal effects. I was hoping their curiosity and the promise of finding treasures in the house would persuade them to get involved. After writing and rewriting the letter a number of times to be sure it was just right and they would not be offended *(Is this possible when evicting someone?)*, I finally sent it to both of them with a copy of my POA.

My patience and energy were wearing thin. I was taking care of my father in my home. I was running into problems in every direction. Things were not going as easily as I had expected. And on top of all of this, there were just too many details to take care of!

Mardig had been writing checks to an official-sounding organization claiming to preserve social security and Medicare. He was sending checks in response to their official-looking documents. David discovered Mardig's *yearly* donations increased to *monthly* and then even *biweekly* payments over the years. We had to put a stop to this. Perhaps it was my naiveté, but I was surprised the organization kept cashing his checks. To our knowledge, Mardig's social security and Medicare benefits were never threatened.

Eight months before arranging to sell Mardig's house, I asked him what he would sell it for if either my sister or brother wanted it. *I considered buying it. I was raised in the house. But I lived too far away and had no plans of moving back to Milwaukee.*

The house was part of Milwaukee's rich history. It was a two-story, red brick Colonial built by a banker in 1923. We found the original blueprints, materials specifications sheets, letters from the original owners, and more in an old dust-covered box in the corner of the attic. I was impressed to see the care given to the selection of materials for the house:

> The mason to furnish and put in the terrazzo finish floors in the front entrance, sunroom, and bathroom, to be of the best grade (guaranteed) . . . must be put in by thoroughly competent and skilled craftsmen in the art of terrazzo-floor laying. Living, dining room on

the first story, and the entire second story . . . finish floors to be 7/8 x 2 1/4" clean oak…white lead and best linseed oil paint to be used for all painting . . . front outside door to be solid oak . . . front entrance transom to be glazed with zincked glass and a cast not less than $2.00 per foot.

Everything in the house was original. My parents were the second owners and hadn't changed a thing. After seventy-five years, the house still had the original boiler, oven, stove, bathtub, sink, and even wallpaper! The inside was generously trimmed in stained solid oak. Even the built-in bookshelves and the majestic mantelpiece were solid oak. The original Edwardian bronze chandelier remained, as did the Edwardian light sconces along the living and dining room walls lined with the original wallpaper. The outside of the house was trimmed with the original copper rain gutters.

My father said, "Sell it to them between five and ten percent below market value."

My sister wanted to buy the house. She said she'd take responsibility for everything inside if she got the house. This sounded like a great deal to both of us! I wouldn't have to deal with clearing out over forty-five years of accumulation and she might find some real treasures! During one of my visits in the spring of 1997, we took time to discuss the details. She said she would buy it.

David called the appraiser and persuaded him to come out the same day. When he walked into the house and began looking around he exclaimed, "This is a museum!" I called a real estate broker and explained the situation. She was willing to do a detailed market value assessment and was generous with her time knowing she might lose the sale if my sister bought it.

My sister's verbal offer was within Mardig's requested range. I gave her a copy of the appraisal. She followed up her offer with a written one. Unknown to me, she faxed it to my computer with a forty-eight-hour response deadline. I had not used the computer in two days when Attorney Cohn called to ask what I was going to do about her offer. *What offer?* After we straightened out my confusion, I went online and retrieved it. I was shocked.

Her written offer was twenty-five percent below the appraisal! *After all our discussions, and all my time, she wasted her time writing up an unacceptable offer.* I called the attorney, explained the situation, and said I would ignore her offer. This failed transaction in June marked the end of our conversations.

We agreed to care for my father. When I signed the POA, I never expected to have responsibility over so many financial details. These tasks took more of David's and my time than the time we spent caring for Mardig. However, as my father's condition worsened and our workload got heavier, David and I began showing signs of Alzheimer's.

THREE

Drowning in Uncertainty

CHAPTER 11

The Ultimate Betrayal

In January 1997, David and I faced a difficult decision. My father's affairs were exceeding the time and energy we had available. Exhaustion was our twenty-four-hour companion. We tried to meet each challenge; sometimes even with humor. Despite our efforts, we couldn't hide our suffering health and depleted energy that was compromising our judgment.

David sent this e-mail while I was traveling on business.

Brenda,

I think I am losing my mind. I could have sworn that I had your father's tax papers, so let me ask you, do I? Or are they in the office closet on top of the box? I'm sorry for asking this, but I swear your father is repeatedly coming into our bedroom at night and I think he may have taken some of his papers.

Last night he got up at 3:30 a.m. and started shaving, he walked around the house for a while, and then went back to bed. I have to be awake to make sure he doesn't turn on any gas. He turned on the gas valve to the fireplace the other day and I caught it right away.

But last night was weird. I was half awake and half asleep, and I KNOW that something got on the bed with me. It seemed like it was the size of a cat, but at the same time, it was like someone or something was patting me, trying to figure out what the shape of my body was. I clearly remember my thoughts while this was happening: This has happened to me many times before. I wasn't scared at all. I also remember thinking whatever was on me or feeling me had the ability to make me immobile—I truly could not move although I was aware. I remember trying with all my might to get whatever it was off me. It was like a contest of wills.

I won! But I broke free with such a force that everything on the bed went flying across the room.

After this happened, I was so convinced something or someone was by the clothes' valet that I grabbed the flashlight to see. Of course, nothing was there. But I know something was on the bed. I would bet my life on it. I am starting to wonder if your father is moving stuff without me knowing it (and without him knowing it too).

I just wanted to share this experience with you because it was bothering me all day and probably will for the rest of the week. Now, I can't find what I did with the tax papers. So, I am starting to think I have Alzheimer's.

Three days later, David sent me the following e-mail. Sally was helping take care of Mardig and she had invited David and Mardig to dinner.

Brenda dear,

Dinner at Sally's was nice. Except Mardig was ornery during dinner. He said he wanted something to eat after he finished dinner but wasn't going to tell me what he wanted. He said I had to figure it out for myself. It was bread. He said he needed bread with his soda. He really likes soft white Wonder Bread. Amazing!

When we got home, he wanted to go straight to bed. While I was helping your father get ready for bed, I heard a noise in the living room. I knew the cats had just finished eating; so, I thought the noise was them. I ran into the living room because I knew Sev would try to pee on the drape. I forgot to lift my foot up over the concrete base of the fireplace and heard a loud crack in my foot. My middle two toes are now swollen, and I have trouble walking.

So let's see, I live in a house with three cats who will try to pee on anything when a human is not in the room, one 86-year old who gets lost in the house, who can't see very good, can't think very good, and can't hear. Now, I'm a cripple and I have to somehow supervise all the 'animals' in the house (at all hours of the day), then I have to drive 83 miles to work and come home and hear the same group of 20 questions about 30 times.

Boy, life is wonderful, and I feel EXCELLENT! I say this all in humor. I am getting by OK.

Love, David

The following day, David went to the doctor to have his foot x-rayed. The crack he heard was a bone breaking. He was given a special shoe to wear and told it would take six weeks to heal.

I wasn't doing much better.

My father had a doctor's appointment, and I was going to take him. We got into the car and I reached over to help him put on his seat belt. My mind was focused elsewhere. *What am I'm forgetting? Do I have all his paperwork for the doctor? I hope we don't have to wait long in the waiting room. The last time, he spoke loudly and even swore. He never swore before. There were children in the room. They looked at us.* I turned the key in the ignition—starting the engine. *David and I will have to make time to review Mardig's bonds to see which bonds have stopped earning interest before year-end. Then again, he may have to pay too much in taxes already. Maybe we'll wait to cash in the bonds until next year. I'll ask the accountant. Oh, geez, I should have brought the papers for the accountant.* I shifted into reverse. *When will this end? I really need to get on with my career! This is no way to build a business. How long can David and I last like this, with so little sleep?* Then I started backing up.

Thoughts swirling around my mind like a blender . . . *BAM!* I stopped. I wasn't going anywhere. *Damn! I had backed into the garage door!* "Oh, shit!" I said aloud.

Mardig looked at me. "What was that?"

I pulled the car forward, hit the remote control to raise the garage door a little to vent the exhaust, and got out to survey the damage. It was noticeable, but nothing that needed immediate attention. "I drove into the garage door," I answered.

"Why?"

I had to laugh! He asked why with such innocence, as if I had done it intentionally.

"Because I wasn't thinking."

"Hey, you're driving, keep your head about you."

He always said "Keep your head about you" when we faced a challenge or when we were overly excited or nervous.

I finished raising the garage door and backed out. Hitting the remote to close the garage door, I noticed it was slightly bowed. Ignoring it, we headed to his appointment.

How stupid! Boy, David's going to ask me some questions.

On another occasion, when I was alone except for a mind filled with distracting thoughts, I backed out and *BAM!* I did it again! I turned off the car and slowly opened the garage door a little, stopping it before it was fully raised, to assess the damage. The damage to my pristine Miata convertible's exterior was now noticeable. It had to go to the body shop. The garage door looked worse. I wondered if I raised it further would it collapse. Then I smiled with anticipation. *This would be a good excuse to get a new metal roll-up door.* I got back into the car, started the engine, hit the remote, and started backing out when I noticed it was getting darker. The door was coming down! I stopped, hit the remote again, and then backed out. CRACK! I backed out too soon. *There goes my power antennae! And what's that noise?* The garage door was making loud creaking sounds. *Okay, one new garage door, one back-end repair, and one power antennae that needed to be replaced . . .*

Mardig had started a new habit. He'd try to open his car door while we were moving. David and I wondered if it was because my car is small and sits close to the ground. Maybe he thought he could simply get out. We agreed I would take David's car when my father had a follow-up appointment at the Center for Aging Research and Evaluation. Sure enough, I did it again. *A second power antennae and the first dent in the NEW garage door.*

We weren't the only caregivers who were losing their minds. Paul almost burned down his house. During one of our caregiver support group meetings, Paul shared the following personal experience:

> My wife likes ham and beans. I was preparing some in a large Dutch oven to take with me when I visited her in the convalescent home. Leaving the ham and beans on the stove, I went to a restaurant to have breakfast. While eating, I heard sirens and saw fire trucks race by. I wondered whose house was on fire.
>
> I finished breakfast and headed home to pick up the ham and beans to surprise my wife. As I approached, I saw a lot of emergency vehicles on my street. I drove forward until I reached my house and realized they had come to *my house!* I wondered what happened.
>
> My neighbor came by and explained. He heard my fire alarm go off and he called the fire department. They came in through the back; I had left the patio door unlocked. They found the stove still on and the ham and beans cooked to a crisp in the Dutch oven.
>
> Stupid me! I had left the stove on when I went to breakfast!

David and I were only in our late thirties, yet we feared we had early-onset Alzheimer's. How else could we explain our behavior?

Things had to change. We would not survive much longer if we continued at this pace. It was time to look at our options and to decide what was best. We considered three.

First, we could purchase a bigger house. My uncle suggested David and I use what was left of my father's assets to buy a large comfortable home for the three of us. Mardig had mentioned getting a place of his own when he arrived in California.

However, a member of our caregiver support group bought a large home with her mother's assets. As the disease progressed, her mother grew increasingly abusive. She and her husband felt trapped but obligated to care for her mother because they were living in her house.

And there is also the uncertainty of how my brother and sister would react. We could buy the house with my father, but we had been careful to keep our funds and Mardig's separate so there would be no perception of impropriety. Plus, David and I didn't want to buy a house. With the fickleness of the real estate market, it would not be a wise investment.

Although a larger home could accommodate a full-time live-in caregiver, we'd need someone at least sixteen hours per day. One person could not work this many hours, so we'd need to hire several caregivers to work in shifts. *Do we even know how to determine who's qualified? Do we have the time to find qualified people? And what about worker's compensation, taxes, etc.? This was getting way too complicated for two exhausted people.* We could turn to a home health care agency, but the costs would be higher. And we still wouldn't be certain of the quality or dependability of the help. What if David and I were out of town and the caregiver didn't show up?

Option two was to place Mardig in a board and care home. The homes we visited had a care-giving couple that lived onsite and cared for a handful of residents in their large home. We liked this personal approach. *But what about the occasional abuses, or the neglect?* We could monitor this with unannounced visits. *But how could we be sure?* Still, this looked like an attractive option: a warm and comfortable home with a family atmosphere.

We were lucky; a nice family had a board and care home in our neighborhood. At the time we visited, they were caring for incapacitated elderly females. My father would not fit in. In addition to being the wrong gender, he still wandered and could easily get over the four-foot-brick wall that surrounded their house. Encouraged by the possibility, we looked for a board and care home where the doors were locked so wanderers like my father could not get out. Apparently, secured doors require special licensing that these homes didn't have.

Our third choice was to consider a skilled nursing home. Once, when Mardig was unbearably ornery, we drove to a nearby nursing home to consider placing him there. We got upset with the idea of him living in an institutional environment. Still, we mulled it over in our minds until we finally found the courage to go inside and ask for a tour. It was very institutional: white walls, sterile environment, and an overwhelming smell of cleaning solution. It was certainly disinfected. Inquiring about the strong smell, we learned the staff was constantly cleaning to keep up with residents who become so disoriented they urinated in the hallways or in their rooms.

How could we pull my father out of our cozy home with plush carpeting, soft recliners, a warm bed with flannel sheets and a down comforter; to place him in a sterile facility with cold tile floors and white bare walls? It was painful to even consider. When we completed the tour, Mardig asked, "Was that for me?"

"Yes," we answered honestly, without thinking, amazed by his candor and fearful he would react negatively.

"It'll be a good place to live once I retire." Hearing this surprised us and gave us some comfort. After all, we justified, he would have twenty-four-hour care in a state-licensed facility. This should ensure enough supervision and no chance of abuse.

One option we couldn't consider was an assisted living community, because they were too far away. We wanted Mardig close to us in case of an emergency. Yet, these communities offered the comfort of home in apartment-style settings with plush furnishings, carpeted hallways, wallpaper, and other touches of home.

When the time came, our best option was the skilled nursing home. David and I had to take a business trip in February 1997, and we needed to be sure Mardig was looked after. Having Jan and Sally care for him during the day was one thing, expecting them to care for him twenty-four hours a day was not an option. Mardig was still taking Aricept®, but he was unable to live independently. *I had hoped Mardig might be the exception and could return home someday, even though the information we received about Aricept® didn't include anything about improvement.* The pain of this decision was too much. We agreed if the combination of activities at the nursing home and Aricept® improved his condition, we would keep Mardig at home with us. *I remained hopeful.*

We visited the skilled nursing home, talked with the staff at length about Mardig's wandering, and learned their precautions and special handling of new residents. We read, tried to understand, and then complete mounds of paperwork. We agreed on a date to admit Mardig before we departed. We had to be sure this arrangement worked. If it didn't, we might have enough time to find another solution before leaving.

We also bought more clothes for Mardig. The nursing home recommended cotton-polyester blend sweat suits that were easy to get in and out of and to wash. We ordered some nice cotton ones from a catalog. While we waited for these to arrive, we went to the department store and bought him a sweater, and more cotton shirts and pants. This way, he would have enough to change into while they washed his clothes. We bought him athletic shoes so he wouldn't slip, tube socks, new underwear, and hangers. I kept his brown jacket, brown dress pants, and his white shirt at home. Someday he may need them for a special occasion, or I may just want to keep them as a memory of his pre-Alzheimer's days.

We had to label everything. *Where do we write his name? Do we write it so every visitor can see he is a resident of the nursing home and knows his name, or should we be discreet and write it inside his shirt collar and on the inside of the pants waistband? Where should we write his name on his socks? What about his shoes? We'd have to get a light-colored gel ink to be seen against the black leather.* We labeled his clothes in various hidden and obvious places. I felt sorry for my father, a grown man. How humiliating, wearing clothes with your name written on them. Labeling my father's clothes reminded me of when my mother helped me label my clothes for gym class. David printed neat block letters, and I wrote his name with a flourish-like calligraphy. I pretended his name was a designer label and tried to feel pride in labeling his shirt above the chest pocket. Once his other clothes arrived, we would have them professionally embroidered, so he would look classy.

Perhaps we could help Mardig keep a little of his dignity. *The challenge was doing all this when he wasn't looking!*

We had to cross a major hurdle. How would we break the news to him? *First, we moved him out of his home of forty-five years to live with us. Next, we were going to pull him from his soft flannel-lined bed. We'd no longer have special breakfasts and dinners together. How would he react? Would he survive?*

The stress and inner turmoil was killing me. Once again, I began writing in my journal.

JANUARY 24, 1997

A day of emotional highs and lows . . . a lot of emotional stretch . . .

Last night, we heard the hum of Mardig's battery powered wet-dry razor. This meant he was getting ready to go to work. David told him we were going to bed because it was nighttime. Mardig laughed it off, as he does when he doesn't agree. He must have stayed up for quite a bit!

Walked in Mardig's bedroom at 7:45 a.m. He was sleeping. This was unusual . . . but then again he thought it was morning last night. I asked him to get up. He wanted to sleep for 10 more minutes. I told him I had a 9:00 a.m. appointment and it was already 8:32. If he slept for 10 minutes, I would surely be late. He said, "Okay," and I extended my hand to help him get up. He got up without my assistance and said my fingers were too thin, that he would fall if he were to grab my hand. *Hmmm.*

He got ready quickly and immediately asked for his shoes. (This question was grating on us for a while now.)

We left for the Adult Day Care Center. I dropped him off at the door because Ellie was standing outside. She took him in.

At 9:00 a.m. I went to the attorney's office to discuss matters pertaining to Mardig's estate—getting the items in his house appraised, appraisers, gifts, etc. I had carefully sorted my notes and created a list of items in priority order. At $200 an hour, I needed to get in and out of there, quick!

At 10:15 a.m. I went to the skilled nursing home to complete a mound of admission forms. The admissions representative was kind enough to mail the forms to us in advance, and David and I had read each page and written questions/comments in the margins. This way I would be able to address specific issues when I was in her office. I was trying to be efficient. The representative said most family members did not ask so many questions nor notice such detail. (I have Mardig's genes.) Still, the reality of this preparation was too much for me to bear. I was able to concentrate on the paperwork and repress what was happening to my body while in her office. It was shortly before noon after I completed nearly an inch of paperwork. Before leaving, I met Mardig's future doctor and we talked for a few minutes. Then I walked outside and my body began to shake.

I lost my sense of orientation. I couldn't think. It was after the noon hour and I needed to go west to the office supply store to buy paper. I froze. I didn't know where to go. It never occurred to me to look in my calendar to see what was next on my list. Those who know me know looking in my calendar is as natural as breathing. I called home and checked for messages. None. I headed south to the credit union to transfer some of our savings to our checking account and to withdraw some cash.

On the way home, I felt relieved I had taken care of Mardig's affairs with the attorney and the skilled nursing facility. I knew in my heart I was doing everything I possibly could for him. I knew someday everything would be scrutinized because of the precarious relationship between my siblings and me. I was determined to do the best I knew how, based on the expert advice I received so I could stand up and defend my actions.

Yet, the future holds unexpected surprises and uncertainties . . .

I had been periodically videotaping Mardig. With his imminent admission into the skilled nursing facility, I wanted to capture as many moments as I could with my father. It was Sunday morning. We were waiting for Dave and Jan to arrive to watch the Green Bay Packers football team *win* their third Super Bowl championship. It would be four to one; four former Wisconsinites against the former Pennsylvanian, Dave. Mardig was reading the Sunday paper at the dining room table while trying to shoo away Djermag, our white cat, who shares his affinity for newspapers. Mardig likes to *read* them. Djermag likes to *roll around* on them.

I stood quietly and zoomed in on my father trying to poke Djermag with the eraser end of his pencil. She'd roll away from him. He gently poked her some more. She turned and swatted at him. He quickly moved his hand back. This went on for a couple minutes until he turned and noticed I was filming him. We laughed.

MONDAY, JANUARY 27, 1997 (5:29 A.M.)

I could not sleep any longer. David left at 4:29 this morning in order to put in more hours so we could admit Mardig to the skilled nursing facility together on Thursday. Thoughts raced through my mind about the day.

Last night, David and I lay awake discussing our feelings and thoughts about telling Mardig.

"So, what do you think, should we just tell him?" I asked.

"Yeah, we have to."

"I agree. We've always been up front with him. But what will we say?"

"We'll just tell him."

"Okay, but *what* will we tell him? I mean, will he even understand? Boy, I feel so awful trying to plan like this, as if it's us against him. Why can't we just explain it to him?"

"Because he doesn't understand."

"When should we tell him?"

"The day before."

"David, we can't wait 'til the last minute! That would be unfair."

"Well, he won't remember anyway."

"Yeah, but waiting until the last minute would be mean. What if he refuses to go?"

"He can't."

"Oh yes, he can. Even though I have a POA, he still lives in America and has rights. Seriously, what if he doesn't want to go?"

"We'll worry about it then."

"But we're leaving in a couple weeks!"

"Well, if it's a problem, I just won't go."

"Will you stay home from work to care for him?"

"If I have to. Otherwise, we'll see if Sally can help us."

"Let's tell him tomorrow night when you get home from work."

"Okay."

"So, what are we going to tell him? You know if [my brother] were here right now he'd say, "Hey, Mardig, you're going into a nursing home.""

David laughed. "Well, it's true, he is, isn't he?"

"But we can't tell him that. He might not understand and get upset."

"He'll forget after a few hours."

"No, he won't. You know better. He remembers feelings and emotions. He may forget why, but he'll remain upset. He may stop listening to us altogether."

"He doesn't listen to us now!"

"Yes, he does. Just not when it comes to removing his shoes . . ."

". . . or going to bed at night," David interjected.

"Well, he might even start asking lots of questions, and repeat them. Do you want that?"

"He already does that!" David said, raising his voice.

"Shhh, we don't want him to come in here."

We went back and forth like this and then lay quietly, trying to drift off to sleep. My body was exhausted, my mind was tired, but my thoughts wouldn't rest.

"David, you awake?"

"Yeah."

"You know, a couple staff members at the nursing home suggested we say he's being admitted in order to be under a doctor's observation."

"Sounds good."

"I suppose it's true, he'll be under a doctor's observation while he's still on the drug study. I wonder what will happen. I need to talk with them to see if his moving affects their requirements for staying on the study."

"Call them tomorrow and ask."

"I will. Hey, how about this: Since you're on the experimental drug study, you need to be under a doctor's supervision for a while. Also, you'll be involved in activities that may improve your abilities."

"Uh-hmmm."

"David, are you sleeping?"

"No . . . well, maybe I drifted off a . . ."

"We'll probably have to let him know we're traveling for two weeks, and we want to make sure he's being cared for—that his meals will be prepared and his other needs will be taken care of."

"Okay."

"Does this mean *you'll* tell him?"

Silence

"David?"

David's asleep. He'll need to get up in a few hours. My body wanted to sleep but my mind wouldn't let it. I lay awake, a prisoner of my thoughts.

"David, you awake?"

"Uh-uhh."

"I'm thinking, what if he doesn't like it?"

"He will."

"How do you know?"

Silence

David got up and showered and I lay awake, my mind still swirling with questions. What other items did I need to add to Mardig's resident contract to make sure all his needs were taken care of? I needed to reread and write notes on the six-page resident rights document. Which clothes and personal items should I bring with us when he's admitted Thursday? I'll have to take some of them to the cleaners so he looks nice at the nursing home. Which friends should I call who would visit him while we were away?

Sigh. This is all for now. Time to make some coffee.

WEDNESDAY, JANUARY 29, 1997

I woke up early and started working at 4:50. Lots on my mind, stomach in knots, acid burning. Took Rolaids® to relieve the acid indigestion. From the separation anxiety of losing a family member, to other issues with people whose behavior and decisions I was trying to understand.

Mardig and I greeted each other at about 5:00 a.m. after I heard his hearing aid whistling. The high-pitched tone had awakened David and me many times during the past months. Mardig would take out his hearing aid and leave it turned on. If something were placed near it, the feedback would cause it to whistle. When I went in his room to turn it off, I noticed he was up. I encouraged him to go back to bed. To my surprise, he said, "For you, I will." *Why do you have to be so sweet and cooperative the day before you leave us?* I tucked him under the covers.

I went into my office to start working.

He got up shortly afterward to go to the bathroom. He came into my room and asked the formidable question that wreaks terror in David's and my hearts, "Where's my shoes?"

Once again, I encouraged him to go back to bed after we talked briefly. He declined, saying he'd rather stay up since he'd already been to bed several times before. He went to the living room and sat on the recliner.

I resumed my work. I had looked for an e-mail from my sister last night and again this morning. I had sent her an e-mail explaining the situation—we were going on business travel and Mardig needed to be watched. I wished she had written something. But there was nothing.

David and I talked about my brother. To our amazement, he had not called. David asked if I would call or contact him. I supposed I should. One of us had to try to behave maturely. Besides, I bet every family has one like him—lives free of rent and utilities, never calls or writes to see how his father is, received a sizable sum of cash via questionable means, claims closeness to his mother while reaping benefits, and then is no where to be found when she dies. But then again, my sister was no different. *How do families get like this? Weren't we raised to be close?* If anyone turned her back, it should have been me! I left at eighteen, never received any help, and never moved back.

I got up to make myself some hot chocolate. I'll drink it to soothe my upset stomach and to warm up. Been having the chills for the last twelve hours! Must be the stress caused by what we're about to do with my father. Then I realize Mardig must also feel like me. I should make him some. This is his second to last morning here. This sends tremors through me. "It's not like he's going to die! It's not like I'll never see him again," I keep repeating to myself. Still, it's a major change for him and us. So, I'll take him some warm chocolate milk with honey. He loves sweet things.

Shall I stay and talk with him? Spend time together? Or shall I continue writing here? I know once he's been away a while, I will have more time, patience, and energy for him. Yet, because he requires so much of my attention and thoughts, his sudden absence will create a major void because my efforts are no longer required.

Time to get his cocoa and talk with him a bit. (6:47 a.m.)

That evening, after torturing myself as to how to tell Mardig he would be living someplace else temporarily, I told him I wanted to videotape him. *For three days, I struggled with how to tell him. I just couldn't bring myself to give him advance notice of where he was going. So here I was, telling him at the last minute. I wanted to capture this emotionally difficult and life-changing moment on tape.*

"Okay," he said.

I was nervous. I didn't know how to begin.

"What do you want me to do?"

"Please, have a seat," I pointed to the rocker and proceeded to set up the camera. He waited quietly until I was finished. I turned on the camera to record and then began asking him general questions about his day.

"What did you do today?"

"I was trying to read the *People's* . . . ugh, *People's* manual . . ."

". . . the *People's Almanac*?" I filled in.

"Yeah."

"So what did you do today?" I asked again. "Do you remember?"

"Really, I didn't do anything. *You* did everything."

"So what did *you* do?" I repeated.

"Well, you took me to the doctor. We got the doctor to say that I'm not falling apart." *He went to the podiatrist.*

"We went to the new place," he continued.

I didn't know what he was referring to, so I asked him another question. "Do you remember what you did at the building behind the church?"

"Yeah."

"Did they throw you a party?" Roberta said they would have a little party for Mardig since it was his last day. I assumed they had, so I tried to jar his memory.

"Nah!" he said chuckling. "They wouldn't throw anyone a party. If I were graduating, I would have to come in the door and throw them a party. On the other hand if I'm just leaving, 'Good riddance. We gotta make room for someone else,'" he said pretending they were talking.

Painfully, I tried to be patient, yet wanted to tell him what was about to happen. I was trying to find a way to smoothly transition into telling him. I just couldn't. I felt tormented. But I tried.

"Mardig, doesn't it interest you . . . it's your last day . . . do you wonder why?" I asked awkwardly.

He started coughing and said, "When you say 'your last day,' keep in mind what you mean . . ." He got up to spit. He returned and continued, "When you say, 'last day' . . . I don't get what you mean 'last day.'"

I didn't know what to say. I felt so uncomfortable. "Well, you know how you've been going to the center every day. Every day you've been going to the center . . ." *We never called it the Adult Day Care Center.*

"Yeah . . ."

"And today is your last day."

"How's that?"

"Because tomorrow you're going to start another thing," I said, being evasive. I didn't know how to say what needed to be said.

"The what?" he asked. Even with his hearing aid, he constantly questioned what he heard.

I repeated, "Because tomorrow you're going to start something else."

"Oh, that's interesting. Tell me about it," he said. "I may not like it, but tell me." *This last comment didn't make it any easier.*

"Well, I hope you like it," I tried to be as enthusiastic as possible. "Uh, tomorrow you're going to be going to the . . . hold on a moment, I want to do something." I had to make sure there was enough tape left in the camera. *What an awkward time to have to stop. It was hard enough getting to this point!*

He began to hum as he watched me. (He hummed when he was happy or nervous.) Then he broke the awkward silence, "A little while ago when you said . . . ahhh . . . as close as we are . . . sometimes, I don't . . . hey, she's a girl!" He looked at David who had just joined us.

"Yeah! Yeah!" I said agreeing with him. "I'm a girl." *He had been having difficulty recognizing my gender. He routinely commented on how cute I was, that I would have no trouble finding a partner. He even tried to match me up with female staff members and volunteers at the Adult Day Care Center.*

"That never occurs to me, there's a difference there. Let's keep the difference . . ."

I humored him. "She has girl parts and you have boy parts," I said.

"That ought to make it even, huh?" he joked.

I was trying desperately to tell him about how his life was going to be different starting tomorrow. I continued, "So tomorrow you begin another phase of your life. Tomorrow we will take you to a place where they will observe you . . . there will be doctors who will observe you."

There, I said it, just the way the nursing home staff suggested. They also advised we tell him he'll be there for one or two days. While he's there, the staff will tell him he'll be there for one more day. They'll keep adding a day until we return or until Mardig doesn't ask anymore. I felt so sad. I was betraying him. There he sat so trusting, so innocent, so helpless!

I mustered the courage to continue. "Remember when we put you on that experimental drug study?"

"Are we done with that?"

"No, that'll keep going for a while."

"The little white, the . . . well we still have that. I got some today, even," he said.

"No, yesterday, last night you got some," I clarified needlessly. I tried hard not to show my discomfort.

"Well, it's a continuation of that, in other words, it's the same level of whatcha m'call . . ." he volunteered. He was making this easier on me.

Why should he? I was betraying him!

"Well, this is a place where you will stay in residence, you'll spend the night there."

"Oh?"

"It will go across several days."

"Oh!"

"And you'll be part of daily activities. There's a large staff there, and they will take you through daily activities. The hope is . . . keeping you stimulated and continuing this experimental drug study . . . that perhaps there might be some improvement." *My brain was working like a wet noodle. Yet, if I stopped talking I knew I would fall apart. I had to get it out. He had to hear what I needed to say. I was betraying him and, if I could keep talking, maybe somewhere in my words, there would be something he'd like.* "The reason why we're doing this at this time is because David and I will be leaving town for a little bit."

"Oh really, how long will you be gone?"

"Two weeks," I emphasized, "and we're going to have to make arrangements for someone to look after you while we are away." *How could I have said this?*

"Child of the house, you mean," he said with a nervous chuckle.

His hand covered his mouth. During the entire conversation, except when he gestured, he covered his mouth with his left hand. This was unusual for him. He usually let his arms and hands rest on the arms of the rocking chair.

"Well, not really, but because you're disoriented we need to help you."

"No, don't . . . don't . . . I understand," he tried to let me off the hook.

"Are you aware of it?" I wanted to know if he knew he was disoriented.

"No, I don't know what you said, but there's a difference when you . . . ahhh . . . reach a certain stage . . . first you're a kid. I treat you as a kid; you're nobody. I mean, I can be impersonal with you and you're supposed to take all that and then suddenly you don't talk with her . . ."

"Well, you haven't said anything inappropriate," I volunteered. When he saw me as a man, he would comment on the appearance of women, and then play matchmaker.

"Well, I . . ."

"You're a diplomat," I added. "You were one when I was a little girl and you continue to be one." I wanted to compliment him. "I just wanted you to be aware. You'll stay at this place and they will evaluate your progress. In February, a specialist will come from Granada Hills to evaluate you. When she . . ."

"She?"

"Yes, she'll be coming up. When she comes up, David and I will be out of town, so you have to behave," I joked.

"Well, it's hard to say if I disbehave [*sic*]! Well," he chuckled mischievously, "I'll be acting like any other *he* person," he said, emphasizing his male gender.

"All men are alike, right?" I was feeling less anxious.

"Right," he agreed.

"I just wanted you to know because it will change your life for a bit. You've been spending nights with us, but because they will be observing you, you will not be spending nights with us."

"Oh, where will I be?"

"You'll be just four miles from our house."

"Oh," he said, his hand still covering his mouth.

"Can I walk that?"

"No, we'll come."

"Well, I can handle that, especially when it's not raining."

This was all I wanted to discuss about the following day with him. I switched subjects and tried to get him to answer some simple questions regarding his awareness. This would be a good benchmark before the disease progressed further.

"Do you know what state we're in?"

"Now, we're going to get into trouble," he chuckled and looked at David. We had discussed this many times during the past weeks. He just couldn't believe he was in California.

"Well, what state are we in?" I repeated.

"Geography says," he chuckled, "name."

"What side of the country are we in?" I tried to make it easier on him.

"On the east side of the country," he replied.

"In what state?"

"New York."

"We're on the east side of the country in New York?" I inquired for clarification.

"Quite a bit of New York is in this part of the country . . . well the fact that I have a bank there that's still on the water and it hasn't moved . . . last I heard I still have the same name."

I switched the topic to his family. "How many children do you have?"

"Oh, this gets to be big," he replied, looking at David and then back at me.

"No, how many children do you have?"

"Three of them," he said confidently.

"What are their names?"

"[My brother's name] . . . ahhh, what is the duke's name?"

I didn't know to whom he was referring. "How many boys? How many girls?"

"Three boys and one girl," he said quickly.

"That's four," I said. "Earlier you said you had three kids."

He hesitated.

I tried again. "How many children do you have?"

"You're one . . . Brenda. There's one a little further north of us and there's another one that I've got a very casual relationship with him . . . I don't think I've even seen his face."

"What are your kids' names?"

"Brenda," he said.

"What's the middle child's name?"

"Uhhh."

"Your daughter . . . you have two daughters and one son."

"And one son?" he asked. "Hey, what did you do with the other son?" he smiled.

"You've never had another son. At least, let me put it this way, in all the years I've lived in that house I never knew of another son of yours. Now, if you have another son on the side, I'll turn off the video camera and we can talk about it."

We giggled.

"Is that a video?"

"Yeah, we can watch it later . . . you can see yourself on TV." I had to repeat things frequently and keep my comments brief since he had trouble hearing.

"Really look foolish, huh?" he said.

"Nahhh, why did you say that?" I inquired. *I was just starting to feel less awful about what we were about to do to him and then he says this.*

"Sarcastic," was his one-word answer.

"Oh."

"Disgruntled and unable to man yourself," he added.

Our black cat, the one who likes to cuddle, came into the room. I picked her up and placed her on his lap. A pleasant distraction, I hoped. He didn't want her to sit on his lap, "I don't want that stranger here." He feared our cats would relieve themselves on him.

"Whose idea is this, all yours?" he asked out of the clear blue.

"What?"

"To straighten me out."

How do I answer such a direct question? "I'm trying to see what can happen for you because I think you might enjoy . . ."

"Well, I may have some female tactics in me."

This took me by surprise. "Explain," I said.

"Childish, let's say."

"You do? Inside of you?"

"Yeah, well because my freedom has generally been with females and since you were also part of the family and very close and also a female, the fact that you were female was completely erased off of you and . . . you male."

"Well, I'm trying to find ways to help you improve if possible . . ." I said, not understanding the point he was trying to make.

"I don't object," he interrupted.

". . . it would be good if you can. You see; the disease of Alzheimer's is a disintegrating disease. But . . . there are drugs and certain therapies to help you improve a bit. There are places with more activities than we can provide. You come here and read, but you don't get enough stimulation, walking around and . . ." *I was making as little sense as he was!*

Our black cat came in again and jumped on his bed. I drew his attention to her.

"Get off of there," he demanded. She ignored him.

"Ohhh, look at the kitty cat," I teased.

"Get off of there," he repeated.

"Nahhh," I teased some more. "Look at her curl up so comfy on your soft fluffy covers."

Our white cat came in and headed for his closet. Our cats had distracted us. I stopped the video camera.

I felt better than I would have had I not said anything at all. Still, I was misrepresenting the situation to my father. Sure, I was told, it was for his own good. Nevertheless, I knew what I was doing and it didn't feel right.

David and I did not sleep that night. Mardig, on the other hand, slept soundly. We didn't hear him get up. I wanted to videotape everything the following morning, but I was so tired and nervous about what we were going to do I didn't want anything to mess up an already difficult situation. I did, however, manage to videotape a brief portion of David shaving Mardig. He dressed himself, but had not shaved, so David carefully shaved Mardig's face as I made stupid comments, trying to detract from my feelings of awkwardness. The tape, at least, will provide us with a warm and touching video of a son-in-law helping his father-in-law.

THURSDAY, JANUARY 30, 1997 (4:25 P.M.)

Well, we did it . . . we took Mardig to the skilled nursing facility. We arrived at 9:00 a.m., one-half hour after our appointment. He walked in willingly; following a few paces behind us, as he frequently had over the past few months. The social services representative pleasantly greeted him with a big smile and asked Mardig if he would come with her. He walked with her through the double doors.

We watched as he crossed the threshold, *the threshold* . . . the locked doors through which he cannot pass until someone signs him out and escorts him. Wow, what a transition in our lives—his and ours!

It was difficult. I had agonized over this decision for the last two days—didn't eat, couldn't sleep, was upset emotionally, and even had diarrhea. David wasn't feeling all that well either! But now, with Mardig admitted, I began to feel better.

It was a *passing* of sorts. He had passed from one place in his life to another. My feelings were even stronger about this transition than the uncertain move from Milwaukee to California.

Now Mardig is in a skilled nursing facility and he thinks he's here under observation for only a day or two. The social services director, who was quite pleasant and charming, assured us this was okay, that the staff will gradually stretch out this observation period. This seemed deceiving. Yet, for a person with Alzheimer's, it is all they know. It is sad. The ultimate betrayal.

Jonathan and Patti were there to visit their spouses and to give us support. I had told the support group earlier we would be admitting my father on this day. Jonathan had endured the pain of admitting his wife, Elizabeth, a few weeks earlier. He knew exactly what we were experiencing. Jonathan waved to us from the other side of the door when we arrived. Once we saw him, he offered to take us out to lunch after we admitted Mardig. We accepted. He helped us deal with this difficult step.

Patti told us later she tried to greet us while we were in a closed-door meeting with the social services director. Patti's husband, Ralph, looks so endearingly at her. Actually, today is the second time I've seen him. The special way he looks at Patti is permanently etched in my mind— head tilted, baby blue eyes lovingly open, and a slight smile. It's a look that says, "How sweet it is to see you, my love." I am sure he was a heartthrob. It must have been hard for her to have him admitted two years ago.

The admission process was thorough. It lasted from 9:00 a.m. to 12:45 p.m. I found being detailed (something I inherited from my father) was useful—meticulous notes, plenty of questions, etc. In a way, by asking questions and taking notes I was honoring Mardig. I remember he took detailed notes throughout my childhood. Now, I was doing the same for him. Furthermore, I requested copies of all records kept on him—psychosocial assessment, admission history, etc.

The psychosocial assessment with the social services director consisted of questions about how Mardig lived one year prior to admission to the facility and about his lifestyle during his earlier years. "Reads everything, likes to do things with his hands—mechanical, electrical, functional things," she wrote on the form. "He didn't do as much with the family since he worked a lot." The social services director asked if he had other children.

"Two more," I said.

She asked if they would visit.

"It's unlikely," I said, with some degree of confidence.

Sadly, after writing to my sister of our plans to admit Mardig, I heard nothing, not even an acknowledgment she received the message.

We inquired why these questions were being asked. The social services director told us this information helps establish a benchmark for Mardig's condition upon admission and it stays on record in the event of a lawsuit.

"A lawsuit?" David asked.

"Yes," she said, "family members could insist they visited every day and played an active part in the person's life, while negotiating an estate settlement."

We also met with the nursing supervisor. We had to make a decision regarding Mardig's health care needs. Do we want him to be revived, sustained, etc.? We opted to customize the simple form. Instead of saying a generic yes or no, we opted for CPR in the facility and then, once he was taken to the hospital and the doctor gave his diagnosis, we would determine the degree of life-sustaining measures necessary. *The ramifications of a simple yes or no are amazing! What if his heart stopped for a minor reason and we said no on the form? He would not be revived. If we didn't give him an option, he had no chance, period.*

We came prepared. I vividly remember our discussions about life-saving measures. In the kitchen and in the basement of his Milwaukee home, Mardig would say, "I don't want my life prolonged if the prognosis is irreversible and terminal." Sometimes, he'd be more definite, "If the prognosis is terminal and life support is the only way I can survive, let me die." Regardless of what we felt, this was *his* life and *his* decision as to how to live and when to die. Based on the doctor's diagnosis at the hospital, we would decide whether or not intravenous (IV) treatment, feeding tube, etc. would be compatible with Mardig's desire.

Sally just went through a similar life and death decision for her father. He did not want to be put on dialysis. His kidneys were weak and not functioning. He would live until the toxins, filtered by unhealthy kidneys, overwhelmed his body. Without dialysis, he would die. She struggled with this, because she felt she had sentenced the last member of her family's previous generation to death. When the time comes, I hope to have her strength.

I wondered if my sister and brother could make these decisions. I assume they would not give Mardig's wishes as much consideration as I did. Knowing this gave me strength as my father's lone legal advocate. What we get out of life is what we put into it. *Right now, I'm putting in too much!*

It's 5:43 p.m. David is pressure-cooking lima beans for our southern-style dinner with Lew this evening. I hear the hiss of the steam escaping. I wonder, What's Mardig doing now? I get up and run toward his room. Oh, that's right. He's no longer here!

CHAPTER 12

The Great Escape!

The phone rang. It was the sheriff's deputy. Martin Avadian had disappeared from the facility. *What? Did I hear that correctly?* Only twelve hours after Mardig walked across the threshold into a different life, we received the worst possible news. *Exhausted, our energy reserves depleted from the events of the preceding days and the admissions process that morning, it was almost impossible to believe.*

The deputy had looked for Mardig but could not find him. As reality sunk in, we felt a rush of adrenaline. Our relaxed evening with Lew took on a sense of urgency. With our hearts racing, we mobilized for action. Thankfully, Lew offered to help.

We took a few minutes to plan. *How far could Mardig get?* Lew would take David's cell phone and drive along a certain route, and David and I would take another route. Whoever found Mardig would call the other. I then telephoned the facility, gave them my cell phone number, and told them what we were going to do.

David and I drove in the direction of the nursing home. We looked up and down the streets and in between buildings. Mardig may realize he's lost and start panicking as he tries to find his way in an unfamiliar neighborhood. We met the deputy at the nursing home and talked briefly with the staff and the administrator before departing.

We walked into stores and into a nearby hospital. We described Mardig to people. Some said they had seen him. Two store employees offered to detain Mardig and call us if he showed up. We were sure we would find him quickly, it never occurred to us to bring photos.

Why hadn't the nursing home called us directly—and sooner?

After searching for an hour without any luck, David and I decided to return to the nursing home to talk with the administrator and management staff in order to learn more details. We called Lew to let him know where we were going and suggested he meet us at the nursing home. It would be helpful to have his congenial Southern charm temper what was boiling inside me. *Prior to Mardig's admission, we had questioned the staff about how they handled new residents. We had warned them repeatedly about Mardig's wandering. They assured us they could handle it. WHAT HAPPENED?*

Immediately the administrator denied responsibility and blamed us! *What?* She said Mardig was too high functioning for the facility. *All the time we were filling out forms and answering questions, no one even hinted at such a thing!*

At the end of a highly stressful night, I detailed the nightmare in my journal as soon as we returned home. In addition to possibly needing the documentation later, I hoped writing would calm me down. *I couldn't believe it! They refused to accept responsibility! They were accountable!*

FRIDAY, JANUARY 31, 1997 (12:26 A.M.)

Mardig disappeared! He was last seen at about 7:15 p.m. according to the director of nurses and at 7:20 p.m. according to an Armenian aide who was with him. The aide said she was watching TV with Mardig and speaking in Armenian about the good old days when she went to get some food. When she returned, he was gone. She assumed he went to his room.

The director of nurses said she got the call that my father was no where to be found at 8:20 p.m. The staff discovered his disappearance at 8:00 p.m., when they give out medications and check on all the residents. *Why were we called a little after 9:00 p.m., over an hour after the facility realized he was missing?*

The administrator explained a lot of visitors leave at 8:00 p.m. and Mardig could have walked out with them.

David and I had driven slowly along the main road on the way to the nursing home. Mardig might try to walk home; however, we doubted it, because it was dark and he became easily disoriented. Along the way, we drove behind the church to the Adult Day Care Center. We noticed the lights were on and hoped to see people we knew. We didn't know anyone. We asked if they had seen an elderly man and described Mardig. They had not. *We were shaking with fear. We had done a good thing for my father by bringing him to California and now look at what had happened!* We continued driving along the busy street, carefully looking up and down the side streets. We saw nothing.

When we arrived at the nursing home, we saw the sheriff's car parked in front. We talked with the deputies who responded to the call. We asked them how they conducted searches. They told us when a child disappears they knock on all the doors in the neighborhood and ask questions. We asked them to help us with my father. They refused to look for my father until twenty-four hours had passed and we filed a missing person's report, because he is an adult. "What if the adult has the thinking ability of a child?" I asked awkwardly. They apologized and said they did not have the resources to conduct such a search. *We weren't feeling very confident just then about how our tax dollars were being spent.*

Lew, David, and I departed to continue our search. What should have taken minutes was stretching to over an hour. The longer it took, the more we lost hope. After two hours, we felt like giving up. *He was nowhere. What were we going to do?* Suddenly, the phone rang. They had found Mardig walking in Rosamond. *What? In another county! How did he get way out there?* We called Lew and asked him to meet us at the nursing home. We needed his support.

When we walked in, the administrator and director of nurses were seated in the administrator's office. Upon entering, a strange sensation overcame me. This had been a scary and potentially dangerous experience, yet something didn't feel right.

"I don't know if we can keep your father here," the administrator said. *Just like that. No discussion, nothing!*

I rejected the administrator's position. My mind raced. Armed with a power of attorney, I was responsible for Mardig. The staff had not acted responsibly and had endangered my father's life.

Before Mardig was admitted, the admissions representative and a supervisor explained their security procedures. We were shown doors with built-in 15-second delay mechanisms. When a person first pushes on the door an alarm sounds, 15 seconds later the lock releases, and the door opens. This is just enough time for an aide to reach the door and prevent a resident from leaving. We were told the lobby area was closely monitored, especially while visitors entered and departed. Furthermore, we were assured that for the first two weeks, my father would receive a lot of staff attention until he adapted to and felt comfortable in his new surroundings. Only hours after he was admitted, the staff was telling us how much they enjoyed him and how much fun he was.

There was a breach. We were told no alarms had sounded. How could Mardig leave among departing visitors if there was someone watching at the front desk? Didn't the person at the front desk have to let visitors out?

We heard some visitors knew the codes to open the doors. We asked the administrator about this. She denied visitors had access to the codes. Yet, during three earlier visits, I had seen staff members openly punch in the four-digit code number. They made no attempt to hide it. Imagine all the warnings we're given about covering our personal identification numbers when using automatic teller machines (ATMs) or a telephone calling card. A visitor could easily read the numbers as a staff member punched them onto the keypad. The administrator negated this idea by stating the codes were changed monthly.

After asking about Mardig's wandering and being told repeatedly the procedures and practices followed by the staff, we were assured they were capable of handling wanderers. They told us other residents also wandered. *So what happened? What good are procedures if they are not adhered to?*

The director of nurses said the nurses and aides who were responsible would be written up. *Is she acknowledging fault here?* I said "writing them up" or finding blame was not necessary. Finding the *cause* was imperative, in order to secure the residents' safety. I think the director of nurses drew some comfort from my not wanting to punish her staff. I wanted them to carefully reexamine their procedures and take measures to ensure they were followed. When I mentioned this, the administrator agreed it was a good suggestion; they would look at their procedures again.

The administrator may have sensed I meant no harm, because she surprised us with her candor: "Brenda, it is difficult to manage our staff closely. And it's hard to find quality nurse's aides. I don't care about a lawsuit. We are foremost concerned about the residents' safety." *Hmmm, I had no intention of suing. What point would it serve? This was a problem in following procedures.*

David explained, "When we were considering this place, we were told residents tried to hide in crowds of people to get out. A nurse's aide mentioned there were two or three incidents when residents escaped within their first days here. Prior to admitting Mardig, we were assured the staff anticipated this kind of behavior and was prepared for it."

Just then, the phone rang. The administrator answered the call. The deputies had arrived with my father. We heard loud noises and got up to look. Two aides were escorting Mardig. For such a cold winter evening, he was wearing only a flannel shirt, pants, and his baseball hat. One shirttail hung outside of his pants and one of his pants' pockets was pulled inside out. His skin was cold to my touch and he was irritated.

When I asked what happened, he said, "I don't know what is happening. I asked some people to let me out . . . I had been talking with some Armenians and it was late. I had to get home."

"Where did you go, Mardig?"

"I walked and walked. I was up for two nights, I was out without a jacket . . . the truck . . . it had no heat, and I was cold."

"What truck?" I asked.

"I was walking and walking and walking. I walked everywhere . . . a man saw me struggling on the side of the road and pulled up beside me . . . I looked inside and saw a friendly looking man, so I got in. We went to the place where the situation was occurring."

Mardig didn't want to talk anymore. He was found about 11:00 p.m. I planned to call the sheriff's office to get more details.

The nurse's aides took Mardig to his room to get him settled.

We returned to the administrator's office. She and the director of nurses expressed their heartfelt concern and said one of them would stay up all night with Mardig. The director of nurses said she didn't feel safe without one of them staying.

There was nothing more to say or do. After we said our good-byes, Lew, David, and I sat in our car and talked about what had happened. Lew shared his concern about the administrator's and director's apathy and unwillingness to follow their procedures.

Moments later, we saw them heading toward their cars. Both had their coats on, and their arms were filled with materials. I was surprised to see *both* of them after they had just expressed the need to stay up all night with Mardig. When they saw us sitting in our car (ours and theirs were the only cars in the front parking lot), they approached one another and talked for a few minutes, then the director of nurses drove away. The administrator walked back inside. Lew, David, and I talked awhile longer, and then Lew walked over to his car and we drove home.

Later that morning, after a few hours of restless sleep, I tried to sort my thoughts. *I couldn't believe the administrator had the nerve to suggest my father should leave. After everything we just experienced, the forms, the questions, the tour, and the options we reviewed; no, this was the best place for Mardig right now.* I had to make sense of what was happening. I couldn't stop feeling nervous. I was under so much stress I could not eat or sleep. I was exhausted. I had an incredible urge to document everything, just in case there was a lawsuit.

I took time to record the following on the computer. As I wrote, more details came to mind. My neck and shoulder muscles tightened as I typed quickly, trying to document everything. I was to suffer many head, neck, and shoulder aches.

FRIDAY, JANUARY 31, 1997 (10:41 A.M.)

I sit here pondering, "What are my rights?" I phoned the attorney and left a message for him to call me. I needed to know my legal rights in this particular situation.

I also called a representative at CARE, to report this incident—a requirement for the drug study. She was surprised and concerned. "What are you going to do? Are you able to trust the nursing home? They should know how to deal with people who have Alzheimer's." She added, "They should have realized this was his first day and he would try to find what was familiar." (Mardig apparently told the nurse's aide he wanted to find his children.) The CARE representative said she would call the nursing director.

I took time to think about what outcome I wanted. Management needed to review their policies and adhere to them. They told us they had ways of dealing with residents who want to leave—for example, distracting and then redirecting the woman who bangs and shouts loudly as she tries to get out the front door. So why did they not see my father leave? The administrator explained yesterday, "If a nurse's aide is preoccupied on the telephone with a personal matter, she will not see Mardig leave." *What does this say about accountability? I can't accept this!*

I want to know steps are being taken to follow the procedures the nursing home already has in place. I want regular updates of the progress being made to follow these procedures. This is all I ask. I am not interested in suing, because I don't believe that would solve the problem. I just want the staff to follow procedures. *Let's get on with caring for the people who, through no fault of their own, have a disease wreaking havoc with their minds!*

10:49 A.M.

I don't want to but I am going to call the nursing home. I want to know how Mardig is doing.

11:14 A.M.

I'm keying these notes into the computer while I wait on hold after being connected to one person, then another. I'm waiting to talk with the director of nurses. I briefly talked with the administrator about Mardig and inquired as to her knowledge of any residents leaving. She said she worked in health care for twenty-one years prior to being the administrator of this facility since it opened. She denied knowledge of any resident actually leaving.

When I asked what she observed about Mardig, she said she does not have medical experience and will defer to her director of nurses. She volunteered that she called and talked with Roberta at the Adult Day Care Center. She reiterated her concern for the safety and appropriate care of the resident. Despite her comments, I am left with the nagging feeling she does not want to accept responsibility for their policies and procedures.

The director of nurses picked up the phone and said she talked with Mardig this morning because he was asleep last night when she went in to see him. (The administrator said the same thing.) Mardig told her he had a son who lived out of state, who was married and had kids. He had a daughter, Brenda. He asked her how far back she wanted him to go when she asked him to tell her of his past. He knew he was born in Armenia. Her assessment was he is relatively high functioning for the facility. The administrator echoed this concern, wondering whether the placement was appropriate. *A fine time to wonder!* She added she would call the ombudsman and the State Licensing Board regarding this situation. The director of nurses then placed me on hold to take another call.

I hate being on hold, it's such a waste of time. Given the circumstances, I held for five minutes, when she finally returned. She said she just spoke with the CARE representative but didn't give any details.

She was rushed to go to an 11:30 meeting. When I offered to call back, she said, "No," and asked me to continue. I did, but I sensed her lack of attentiveness. *She was simply going through the motions.* I asked if the code numbers had been changed. She said she didn't know; that was the administrator's department. *It was strange she would brush aside one of the major issues we discussed the night before.* I asked her if she punched in the same code she punched in yesterday, and she hesitatingly said, "Yes."

I repeated what I suggested to her and the administrator the night before: "Changing the code would be the first step to improving security." She said she'd relay my message to the administrator.

As we ended our conversation, she said to call any time if there's anything else they could do. *What a disingenuous attempt to appear polite!*

"Please change the code numbers, that is the first step," I repeated.

She muttered "Uh-huh."

FEBRUARY 6, 1997

This has actually been a living hell! If I didn't care so much, I wouldn't do anything.

Well, that's just it . . . why get into all the formalities, legalities, and regulatory stuff if we don't have to?

So then, here goes . . .

Tuesday the 4th I went to the caregivers' support group meeting at the facility. It was scheduled to begin at 9:30 a.m. The social services director came in at 9:40 and apologized for being late. I listened and observed intently. This would be interesting, helpful. Moments later, the social services director was called to the door by the director of nurses. They spoke awhile, then she returned. At a little after 10:00 a.m. I asked my first question. The social services director asked me if I had any more questions.

I said, "No." *That was weird . . . to be asked such a question in a support group setting.*

She then asked if I had any comments.

I shook my head and said, "No."

"Because you have a ten o'clock meeting."

"Excuse me?" I inquired. *People didn't even know I was planning to attend. How could I have a ten o'clock meeting?* "With whom?"

"There's a gentleman who wants to see you," she said as she stood up. She motioned me to follow her out the door.

I asked, "Who?" By this time I had packed my notebook, gathered the stuff I had brought for Mardig, and rushed to follow her.

I asked again, "With whom?"

She said, "[person's name]."

I inquired, "[person's name]?"

"You don't know him?" she asked, surprised.

"Who is he?"

"He can help you in dealing with these kinds of things." Then she rushed ahead of me down the hallway and I tried to catch up, which was hard with residents ambling through the hall.

I followed her out the front doors into the administrator's office and there, to my left, seated and looking at the floor, was the director of nurses. To my right was a man standing by the chair where I was invited to sit. He was the corporate attorney.

I was sandbagged! How could they do this to me? And to pull me out of a support group! I tried very hard to retain my composure and didn't think to ask, "Why are you meeting with me—three on one?" I thought of saying I wanted my attorney present; but I didn't. I just wanted a resolution of this frustrating mess created by their irresponsibility.

After the obligatory, but *awkward* introductions and handshakes, I retained enough composure to assert myself: "I will listen to what you have to say and then I will say what I need to. Afterward, I will visit my father and then leave to clear my head."

Not acknowledging what I said, they asked if I received their letter. "No," I said.

"Federal Express was to deliver it Saturday."

I said, "Oh, you were the ones who sent a Fed Ex package! I got a notice from them on Monday the 3rd to sign the release so they could leave the package. I should get it today (Feb. 4th)."

The administrator looked disappointed and said she'd make a copy for me.

As I read the letter, I became numb. I had difficulty focusing on the content. I found myself judging how the letter was written. The first sentence was incomplete. Commas and hyphens were missing. It had not been proofread. Strangely, I gained strength from this.

January 31, 1997

Dear Ms. Avadian,

In regards to the admission of your father Martin Avadian to the [Skilled Nursing Facility] on January 30, 1997.

Because of the incident of Mr. Avadian leaving the Facility on the same night of admission, and planning to do the same today January 31, we feel that we are not able to assure the safety and security of him.

[The Skilled Nursing Facility] is a secured facility for Alzheimer's and others Dementias, and is not a locked facility. Residents retain their right to leave this facility, as in any other long term care facility.

As Mr. Avadian's DPOAHC, and legal representative, please make arrangements immediately for more suitable placement for him. Please inform us of your plans on Monday February 3.

I regret that this placement was not successful, but our main concern is the safety, security, and well being of the resident.

With regards,

[Administrator]

cc: Corporate Attorney

The letter was dated one day after the incident. *So much for coping with people who have Alzheimer's. So much for giving them a chance!*

I was dumfounded! They assumed this placement was "unsuccessful." "Inform us . . . by February 3." I had not even received the letter by then! What a way to wipe their hands clean of their responsibility! I was incensed, yet afraid. I had to learn my rights.

This is an Alzheimer's skilled nursing facility. They know some residents will try to get out during the first few days. The admission's representative assured us during the first few weeks they kept a close eye on new residents.

They screwed up. Plain and simple. They had stated their procedures. They just refused to be held accountable to them. Doesn't make sense!

Before I saw their letter, I had called a few people—the sheriff's station and Mardig's doctor (their medical director), who claimed the placement was appropriate given Mardig's mental ability. Now, I'm calling more—three offices of the ombudsman, deputies of the other county, California Highway Patrol, attorneys, and friends. I wanted to get as much information as I could and to learn my rights. The attorney and ombudsman assured me one of five conditions must be met for the facility to release my father:

1. The nursing home has ceased operations.
2. The resident failed to pay.
3. The resident's presence endangers others.
4. The resident's health has sufficiently improved.
5. They cannot properly take care of the resident.

I also learned of other families' issues with this facility. Despite all this, I wanted my father to remain. It was a clean place, close to home, and it generally provided quality care.

One ombudsman advised me to write a letter and send a copy to the Department of Health Services (DHS). I learned the facility was already being investigated; I didn't want to create any more trouble. After all, where else would Mardig live? When I hesitated, she emphatically asked me to consider what I would do if I turned on the TV and heard another resident had walked out, was lost, and later found dead? How would I deal with that, knowing I could have brought this to DHS's attention, to avoid future occurrences? She added, "A fat fine would be waiting for them since they found your father all the way in Kern County!" I did what I believed was best. On February 6th, I completed my written response to the letter the facility sent to me.

6 February, 1997

Dear [Administrator]:

This letter is to respond to and acknowledge your letter dated 31 January, 1997 and delivered to me by Federal Express on 4 February, 1997 regarding my father, Martin Avadian.

As his Attorney-in-fact, I was assured prior to his admission that [the facility] (herein referred as: "Facility") could handle a resident with my father's needs—e.g., wandering, Sundowner's syndrome. My husband and I have been regularly assured by your staff that you routinely deal with residents who want to *get out* and that you have *creative* ways of handling them.

Upon our expressed concern to your staff regarding my father's wandering and agitation, we were informed that residents have and do try to mingle among visitors near the front door and then leave! We were assured that your staff deals with this and that your policy is to have two staff members at the front desk at all times since residents do try to get out.

Given this, you can imagine the surprise and scare we received when we learned 12 hours after his admission that he could not be found in the facility! Your staff noted he was missing at approximately 7:30 p.m. on Thursday, 30 January, 1997 and we received the call at 9:05 p.m. saying a sheriff's deputy would like to speak to us. Our first thought, given all these assurances we received, *how did he manage to get out?* Yet, when we (my husband and a close family friend) walked into your office, your initial comment was, "We don't think we can keep your father here."

A report filed by the CHP noted that my father was picked up in another county! Imagine that! Due to your negligence to follow your own clearly articulated procedures to insure the safety and security of your residents . . . look what happened to my father. What if another resident got out and was not as lucky as my father? (We have heard from your staff that this happens!)

In spite of this oversight, I desire to keep my father in your facility. He expresses how much he likes it there. He thinks he's been there for several years. Your staff regularly informs us of how much they enjoy him. We have been told that since this initial incident he has not tried to get out. Sure, he, like many of your other residents, will express a desire to go home. Still, we have been repeatedly told that he has not tried to get out.

I would like to be assured that you will follow your procedures—changing the access code (if you have not already done so), asking your staff to keep the access code covered when entering or leaving the facility (similar to when we use ATM machines), and keeping the front desk staffed at all times. You have a very caring staff, I am sure this was as much a scare to them as it was to you and your Corporate Attorney.

I am fully aware of my rights and if we cannot resolve this situation, I will take further steps.

Genuinely yours,

Brenda Avadian

cc: [Ombudsman]

FEBRUARY 6, 1997 (9:46 P.M.)

This is getting tiring. Instead of being able to relax, I need to continue to journal in order not to lose my memory of these things. Why? Because a few people cannot be responsible nor accountable. Such is life. We are all interconnected, what one does impacts many. The staff's oversight resulted in my father's disappearance, leading to the involvement of a lot of people, resulting in management's denial due to fear of accountability and liability. *Life becomes toxic when one points the finger at someone else!*

Mardig called me this morning. He is unaware of the passage of time. Instead of days, he thinks he's been living there for years. He refers to his room as "home." He said, "If you have a couple hours to throw away, come visit me as I would like to talk with you at some length."

He felt awkward talking on the phone, so we started speaking in Armenian. I reminded him he could still speak Armenian and I could understand it, so he could feel free to talk.

In Armenian he said, "They're tiring me ... they are asking me a lot of questions." He said he's doing nothing there, but if his being there is helpful to me, he'll stay. *The unfailing diplomat, even with Alzheimer's.*

He said the staff is friendly, nice, and smiles. He says he keeps losing his pencils and pens. Mardig likes writing notes to himself. Writing short notes provides him comfort, even though he loses the paper he writes on. He advised me to call him a day in advance of my visit so he would be at home (his room), since he tends to wander a lot outside (the halls). He wanted to keep in touch with me just in case I moved or changed my phone number. He wanted to be sure we were "still connected."

Jan called David this evening to apologize for not visiting Mardig. She planned to visit Mardig today. She was afraid the staff would ask her more questions.

She explained last night they took her to a room and asked her many questions. *Who is she? How does she know Mardig?* Then they inquired about David and me. She could not easily recall the specific questions. Nonetheless, before she left yesterday, they asked her for her name and number so they could contact her if necessary. She said this would be fine. Today she felt uncomfortable and could not face their questions. *Why would they question a visitor and nonfamily member in this way?*

FRIDAY, FEBRUARY 7, 1997 (1:41 P.M.)

I visited Mardig today from 10:55 to 11:50 a.m. He was happy to see me. I was a familiar face in a sea of unfamiliarity; someone in whom he could confide. Jan came about 25 minutes after I arrived.

"They're putting restrictions on me," he said. He was trying to get out and they would not let him or gently redirect him. *This was good!* He said he wanted to get out because he wanted to walk around the area. He was used to doing that. I reminded him of the incident when he tried that and found himself in another county. I explained he was lost and the police had to bring him back. He had no recollection of the incident.

I had to leave. Jan said she would stay with Mardig a few more minutes.

Later, Jan called to say that as she was leaving, the social services director said she thought Jan was my father's daughter. *Hmm, this is strange. Just a week earlier, I met with this director for 45 minutes to complete my father's psychosocial assessment.* The social services director asked her to relay a message to me. *Why are my father's visitors getting this kind of treatment?*

SATURDAY, FEBRUARY 8, 1997 (11:15 A.M.)

Jan called and said she just got back from seeing Mardig. When she got there, she said Mardig was lying in bed reading the newspaper. Jan brought a picture for Mardig to stick on the white board that the staff mounted on the wall for us. *Does this mean he can stay?*

Mardig said the picture might be stolen if it was put there, so he placed it in his drawer instead. The picture was of Dave and Jan at a formal event.

Mardig commented on how handsome Dave looked. Mardig also said, "Ma was very busy taking care of the kids, and that is why she doesn't come to visit me." Mardig explained if he lost his job, he would have to get another one to make sure all the bills were paid.

Jan said she just listened to him talk and she didn't really remember anything else he said. She ended her visit when a nurse came in and said he had to take Mardig's vitals. She said no one asked her any questions this time and it was a very pleasant visit.

11:43 A.M. (DAVID'S NOTES)

Our neighbor who cares for our cats called. I told her about the situation with Brenda's father. I keep waking up in the night thinking about Mardig at the nursing home. I wake up thinking about him and go to bed thinking about him. I think about him when I am at work and on my way to and from work. I worry the nursing home won't treat him nicely because they think he's too much trouble. That's all.

Days pass into weeks. David and I take our two-week business trip while Jan visits my father. When we return, there is a letter dated February 14 from the facility's corporate attorney. (We told the facility we'd be away the 11th through the 23rd. Apparently, they are so convinced of their righteousness, they resort to sending mail knowing we won't see it until we return.) The attorney threatens to "institute a formal notice of discharge and transfer" unless we respond immediately. He includes the doctor's opinion: "your father is at risk at this facility" and the CARE representative's statement: "facility is clearly inappropriate . . . your father should be transferred as soon as possible." Furthermore, he writes: "We were visited by the Department of Health following your complaint."

Lies! All lies! I started making phone calls immediately. The doctor told me this place is "the best facility for Mardig given the locale." The CARE representative said they took her comments out of context. *Who can I believe? Everyone tells a slightly different story depending on who is listening.* I never called nor corresponded with the Department of Health, so I doubt the validity of the attorney's comment about them coming to the facility following my complaint.

I call Jan and some of the staff members. My father has been doing well and has not tried to leave. I followed up with the administrator.

She seemed less insistent and we uncomfortably agreed to monitor my father.

As the weeks pass, Mardig seems more comfortable and refers to the facility as his home. We learn he occasionally tries to get out, as do a number of other residents. But as far as he is concerned, he is *home*.

I have not talked with the administrator since, except for a polite hello. I have not seen much of the director of nurses either. I hoped surviving this trauma together would have given us a special bond. Despite all of this, I am satisfied my father is home and the staff is taking good care of him.

We learned the following during these weeks: ask a lot of questions, know your rights, and stand up for them. This skilled nursing home is the best option we have right now.

Note: The skilled nursing facility changed ownership in December 1999. Today, the Antelope Valley Care Center is owned and managed by people who care.

CHAPTER 13

Our Family
Finally Gets Together

I often wonder, When will all of this end? David and I keep hoping the worst is behind us. Since we don't have children, we can only imagine the demanding role of being a parent. But, with children, at least there is usually a future to look forward to. Barring any unforeseen circumstances, children will mature into self-sufficient adults. *Well, this is the way it's supposed to be!*

In contrast, people with Alzheimer's do not grow *up*. In fact, the most caregivers can hope for is to enjoy small gifts, such as a smile, being recognized, and other special moments together. Any of these give caregivers pleasure and enable us to endure. Yet, these simple pleasures are often overshadowed by sizable responsibilities: disposing of loved ones' personal effects, selling their homes, relocating them, organizing their finances, and overseeing their health care.

In April 1997 David and I stood in Mardig's living room, intimidated by the prospect of cleaning out my parents' home. They saved *every-thing!* We faced boxes stacked to eye level. In some places, boxes were so high, we couldn't see above them. While moving a stack of boxes,

David was surprised to discover the fireplace that had been hidden for years!

Upstairs, the once wide-open, bright, and airy master bedroom was cluttered with cartons, stacked from floor to ceiling against every wall, except where my mother's hospital bed stood. The dressing room with two mirrored closets had not been used in a long time; the towering boxes barely left enough space to maneuver around. As we cleared out the dressing room, David exclaimed, "Brenda, I didn't know there was another window in here!"

At the opposite end of the house, my former bedroom was being used for storage. Leaning against the wall, behind piles of more boxes, were a half dozen outdoor windows and wooden shutters. One dresser remained, but the bed had been disassembled and the mattress, frame, and wood supports were leaning against a wall. The door leading to the attic was in this room.

If the first and second floors were intimidating, the attic took us over the edge. It was The Avadian Family archeological site, complete with baby clothes, a five-year supply of toilet paper, a lifetime supply of light bulbs, my brother's belongings, Christmas lights and cards, green industrial light fixtures, and nearly one hundred small wind-up alarm clocks. My mother would go to the outdoor flea market and buy things with the intent of selling them at a profit. *She obviously bought much more than she sold!* We wondered how we were ever going to clean this house. David suggested we go downstairs for a change of venue.

We carefully walked down the steep wooden steps.

My mother stored loaves of bread on these stairs during the winter months since it was cooler in the attic. She'd buy too many; sometimes ten to fifteen loaves a week for our family of five. We'd never eat all of them before they grew mold. My father failed to convince her to buy fewer loaves. She'd say in Armenian, "Never mind, we'll eat them." When we protested about eating moldy bread, she showed us how to tear away the moldy parts and eat the good parts. I learned toasting bread takes away the moldy smell. Once, when my mother, sister, and brother went to the flea market, leaving my father and me home, I persuaded him to dump the old loaves so we could eat fresh bread. He finally agreed and buried several in the garden. A couple months later, while cultivating the garden, my mother discovered the blue printed plastic bags and we had hell to pay. She argued with my father and refused to talk with me for not telling her Mardig had buried the bread!

David and I went into the basement. There seemed to be fewer items, but we soon realized this was an illusion. The three largest rooms of the four allowed everything to be spread out. The smallest room was stacked floor to ceiling with boxes and wooden crates filled with motors, spare parts, wire, plumbing supplies, and more. Mardig accumulated two or three of the same thing; particularly tools. *When he couldn't find something or forgot he had a tool, he'd buy another one.*

I found three treasures that took me back to my childhood. One was an old food scale that could weigh items up to twenty-five pounds. Even though it was not accurate, it was a part of our family history. Mardig said he used this scale to weigh each of us after we were born. When we were older, we used it to weigh the watermelons my mother stored in the cool basement during the summer months. We had contests to see who could guess the watermelon's weight.

The second treasure was a box of Mardig's cameras. I didn't remember all of them, but one I recognized. He would use it to take our pictures at school events, like music concerts. He was the only one with such an old camera and I was often embarrassed by him standing near the stage in the dark auditorium, unaware he was blocking others' views. While my classmates' parents used portable cameras to take photos quickly, my father made a production of it. Dressed in his forties-style double-breasted suits with matching ties *(I went to school in the sixties!)*, he'd take time to set up the tripod, compose his shot, focus, charge the flash, and then shoot.

The third treasure was an old hand-crank meat grinder. Mardig would mount it on the workbench downstairs, lay clean newspaper around it, and then my mother would grind a special cut of beef for *chi kufta*. This is an Armenian appetizer of raw beef mixed with finely ground cracked wheat, green onions, parsley, and cayenne pepper. Since the rest of the family disliked raw meat, my mother and I would enjoy this fine appetizer. She'd say, "In Beirut we'd use lamb instead of beef." And then she'd lift one hand and put the tips of her fingers together and place them against her pursed lips to illustrate how tasty the *kufta* was in the *old country*.

I relished the memories as we walked up the stairs to the sunroom, where Mardig kept most of his papers. Each file folder and envelope had to be closely examined as they were not labeled correctly. Important and unimportant papers were haphazardly mixed together. He frequently hid things. We found documents between pages of old newspapers stacked in the living room. We couldn't assume anything was a pile of junk and just toss it. This process alone took upwards of a hundred hours for the two of us. As soon as we celebrated making it through the bulk of the paperwork, we would find more. We could easily work another hundred hours and still barely make a dent in all of my father's papers.

My parents' belongings had to be sold, donated, or disposed of; then their home was to be sold. David and I met with an estate sale administrator, a cleaning service, a real estate appraiser, and a real estate broker. Each expressed amazement at the amount of stuff my parents accumulated. I heard comments like, "Hope you're not an *only* child." "Wow, I'm not envious of what you have ahead of you." "Good luck!" "Look at these antiques!"

My brother and sister surprised us by offering to help during the last three days. I happily welcomed them. Their presence erased from my mind their lack of earlier involvement. We worked hard to make progress, but there were just too many things to look at. My brother arranged to rent a commercial trash dumpster from the waste disposal company he used for his business. They delivered it on a huge truck and dropped it off in the backyard.

We divided our labor. The girls—my sister, my brother's girlfriend, and I—sorted through my mother's clothes, boxed materials, and sewing supplies in the master bedroom. I was amazed at all the things our mother packed!

She and Mardig wanted to move to a warmer climate along the West Coast. We girls set aside the items to be discarded, then the men loaded them into the huge container in the backyard.

After several hours, we grew emotionally weary of sorting through

Ma's stuff and, for a change of pace, headed downstairs toward the two-car garage with twelve-foot ceilings (plus attic) to see what we could clear out. We carefully walked along the back sidewalk on the slippery snow. I don't remember who started it, but soon we were throwing snowballs at each other. Laughing and running around, I wondered why we couldn't get along better since we did have fun when we spent time together.

The garage was just as cluttered as the house, except the objects were much heavier. On the lower level were wooden crates filled with scrap metal, cardboard boxes stacked atop a trailer, and various-sized cans filled with assorted items—we hadn't yet ventured into the attic. We helped each other lift the heavy crates and neatly piled them along the walls of the walk-in garbage container. The boxes of unopened engine oil from twenty years ago and old pesticides, some containing DDT, were considered hazardous materials, so we disposed of them separately.

With all the heavy lifting in the cold April air we tired quickly and decided to quit for the night. We made time for a fun dinner out, where our energies revived as we relentlessly teased one another.

The following day, we returned to work. After another long, hard day of excavating our parents' things—and discovering enough laundry detergent in the garage attic to supply a small town for a year—we stopped. There was no more room in the trash container. My brother called to have the container picked up and another one dropped off. These dumpsters were huge, measuring twenty-five feet deep by eight feet wide and eight feet tall.

That night we ordered pizza to eat while sharing memories and watching videos of Mardig I brought in anticipation of such an occasion. We also continued to tease each other.

My sister found one of our mother's print skirts with lace trim. She began toying with it around her waist when I grabbed my camera. She quickly held it up to our brother's waist and I snapped a picture before he even knew what happened. We managed to get a few photos of him in compromising situations. He hated having his picture taken, which made it even more fun.

Just as quickly as our excitement escalated, the room became quiet. "Brenda, listen to me," my brother declared.

"What?"

"Are you listening?"

"Yes," I said, looking at him. Everyone looked at him.

"Brenda, you know we give you a hard time and tease you, but thank you for taking on this difficult job."

"Yeah, thank you," my sister chimed in, "for bringing us together." My heart melted. I looked at them dumbfounded and then I smiled. *I hoped we could work and be together again.*

We looked around. There was so much stuff our mother had meticulously packed. We found thirty pairs of scissors, each carefully wrapped in tissue paper and bound with string. What would we do with all of them? We continued sorting and then chose a few items of her clothing to keep as reminders of her.

While going through our mother's dresser drawers, we found her hairnets and silk scarves. Holding them up to our noses, my sister and I drew in her scent. Distracted, I didn't notice our brother had walked out of the room, until I heard sobs from his old bedroom. I didn't know what to think or feel. His girlfriend went to join him. My sister thought he must not have faced his grief over our mother's passing four years earlier and was now overwhelmed among her things. I was temporarily frozen, not knowing how to react. I had never seen this side of my brother. Over the years, I grew accustomed to his hardened, uncaring, and temperamental qualities. I saw him as a man who tried to be in control of every situation. Plus, after years of being encouraged to temper our emotions, we were uncomfortable sharing them. We agreed to give him his space.

The following day, Sunday, April 13, 1997, we gathered in the dining room. This was to be a family conference to discuss unfinished business regarding our father's estate. Issues remained including the sizable funds our brother had obtained under questionable circumstances. All six of us were present, my brother and his girl-friend, my sister and her husband, and my husband and I.

I overviewed the reason for the meeting and asked permission to audiotape our discussion to prevent any misunderstandings later on. My brother positioned the tape recorder so the microphone would pick up all of our voices. After pressing the record button, he stated the date and time, "Sunday, April the thirteenth. Time now, ten-thirty on the head, Central Standard Time." Each person gave permission to be audio taped and stated his/her name for the record.

I was struck by my brother's eager cooperativeness and struggled to restate the purpose of our meeting. I awkwardly started with, "You know, you guys could have done all this . . . handled Mardig's affairs. You're here. It's been difficult . . . David and I live so far away."

"But you both are August twenty-twos!" my brother exclaimed, referring to my shared birthday with Mardig. "Let the record show that, too, Brenda," he said, leaning toward the microphone.

I felt uneasy. Inadequate thoughts of how best to approach the delicate subject filled my mind. "That's okay," I interrupted.

"Yeah, you Augusts always stick together. In other words, it's probably best you do it because you're August, he's August. You two acted the same . . . we referred to you as 'Mardig, Junior.' You have the same mannerisms, you have the same thought process."

I chuckled uncomfortably; wanting to believe this was a ringing endorsement of my duties on behalf of our father.

"Brenda, it's not funny. It was something that even used to grill Ma to no end, sometimes because of the fact that you were . . . uh . . . uh . . . literally 'Mardig Junior.' I don't know how else to explain it. Okay. You acted like him. You had many of the same characteristics. It's not meant to be derogatory, but it's . . ." he paused a moment to catch his breath, ". . . it was best that one Mardig took care of the other Mardig."

This is a ringing endorsement if I heard one! I was strengthened by his words.

"I want to . . . ugh . . . just get back to the financial situation. Is everybody comfortable with an equitable division of the estate?"

"It's fine," our sister said after a couple of inaudible comments.

Our brother volunteered, "[Our sister] has never been . . . you know . . . [she's] never really been aggressive. [She's] got so many of her own headaches, she doesn't want to be bothered with anybody right now."

"And how about you?" I ask.

"I pretty much have the same attitude," our brother answered.

"Okay. The reason I bring this up, is because what happens is, when we look at something of benefit we get caught up in the details and say, 'Well, I want this . . . I want that.'" I felt so uncomfortable! We all did!

"Uh, Brenda?" my sister interjected. "You, number one, did not work for it. You're not entitled to it. This is for them [our parents] to enjoy and if they chose to, you know, do what they did with it [interrupted by a watch sounding an hourly chime], that's fine. We were [inaudible] they benefited us by raising us from zero to eighteen. Their obligation is [inaudible] after that."

"Yeah, I'm glad you said that because that's exactly the perspective we need to maintain through all of this," I said, hoping we could now discuss the key issues.

"Uh-hmmm," she agreed.

"So . . ."

"Yeah, I concur with [our sister]," our brother interrupted.

"So, all right! That's it, I guess," I conclude.

"Okay, now, the other question. All this legal mumbo jumbo with all these schmantzy uhhh high-falutin' doggone lawyers that uhhh, you know, know how to suck you dry . . . okay . . . and that can go right on the damn tape, too. . . . Do we get a copy of all of this? Or are we . . . uhhh . . .?"

"All of what?" I ask my brother.

"In other words, you said you've a lawyer there. Pay attention to me, please, if you would be kind enough."

"I am paying attention to you."

"Okay, but you're writing something down."

"Yes, and I can still pay attention to you."

"No! No! In this case you can't quite do two things at once. Okay, we've got lawyers over here. We've got one there. Hello! Okay, we've got one here . . . who does what?"

"Uh, Mardig retained an attorney to get back the money you have."

"Keep going," he urged.

"Yeah . . ." added our sister.

"Yeah, there's a whole argument there in of itself. But I'm not going to get to that right now," my brother added.

"He retained an attorney here with the sole function of getting back the funds and also because you were trying to get the house. And that . . ." I started to explain.

"And that's where you're going to get a battle on your hands, Brenda. Because the fact of the matter is that when Ma was around . . . okay, back when I was twenty-seven, twenty-eight, I shelled out a ton of money for the house. It was paid to them and paperwork was signed."

"Do you have proof?" I asked.

"Oh, yes."

"Would you like to show it to me?"

"I don't have it on me."

"Okay, if you have proof you wrote out a check and it was for the house and it has been documented, I need to see it."

"Okay."

"Okay?"

"Right, right."

"All right?"

"Okay."

"But let me tell you one thing. The paperwork is incomplete. You guys tried to execute the transfer . . ."

"Uhhh . . . no. Ma and Mardig and I went down there. We paid the money. Once Mardig got the money, then Mardig all of a sudden backed out."

"There is no documentation of such an occurrence," I said.

"Okay."

"And if you need to claim that, you need to produce

documentation because there is absolutely no documentation of . . ."
I was interrupted again.

". . . Well, I've got the paperwork to that effect, so . . ."

"Umm."

"The thing is, though, it was incomplete because Mardig always goes off in his weird areas."

"No . . ." I started to argue

"Mardig . . ."

"It is solidly documented," I cut in. Mardig felt he was being taken advantage of and he drew the line on the house. You need to know the way you acquired the money can be a criminal act."

"No!"

"I am not talking as Brenda, your sister. I am talking from a legal perspective."

"Well, you know, I'll tell you right now. Ma made it quite clear . . ."

"She is not here," I reminded him.

". . . she said, 'I want you to get that money, because once I die, Mardig will not leave you a cent.'"

"You understand what you are saying here. You're talking about Ma and Mardig's estate that is to be left . . . you just said you agreed with [our sister] totally . . . what they worked so hard for . . . why would Ma want to carve out . . . ?"

"Ma wanted her half."

"Listen, why would Ma want to carve out something from their mutual estate and give it *just to you* and have Mardig not have enough to support himself? Does that sound logical?"

"Yes, it does! Because Ma did not want . . . I'll answer that, okay?"
I started to interrupt him.

"Let me answer this!"

"No, this is . . ."

"I wanna answer this!"

"This is extraneous."

"No, it isn't! It is crucial to the matter," he insisted.

"The point is, this is a *community* property state. What is Ma's is Ma's and Mardig's and what is Mardig's is Ma's and Mardig's. And that is their estate. Okay? Hear me. Regardless of what you say, this is *their* estate. We have documentation . . . hear me very clearly . . ."

Our sister coughs.

"Regardless of what Ma said to you, we have documentation that the way you got the money was questionable."

My brother and I went back and forth like this as the tension mounted. David interjected a few times with what we found in Mardig's papers. We came to no resolution.

"Hey," our sister cleared her throat, "it's getting late. If we're going to brunch we should be leaving now." We had agreed to go to Mader's, a fine German restaurant.

Once there, our earlier conflicts vanished. Once again we laughed, teased, and enjoyed each other's company.

We returned to the house afterward, our stomachs filled with delicious German cuisine, and worked until we filled the second trash container. There was still a lot more to be cleared out of the house.

David and I planned to fly back to California the following evening. David had to return to a new job and I was feeling pressure due to lost business opportunities while I was occupied with my father's affairs. I turned down the opportunity to teach a course at the University of Southern California. I was turning down consulting assignments worth thousands of dollars, and I stopped working on my fourth book. One ray of hope brightened our departure: our family being together may mean we'll stay together through the rest of this journey.

CHAPTER 14

Mardig Returns Home

We wanted to bring Mardig home for a visit. The staff advised us not to take him out of the facility too soon. "It could disrupt Mr. Avadian's adjustment to his new *home*," they explained. So we waited. We visited him regularly. Each time we wanted to bring him home, the time was not right. *When would the time be right?*

We grew concerned his health would deteriorate and he may never leave the facility if we waited for the *right* time. Besides, he wanted to go out! He kept asking about going to work, shopping, the bank, and more. David and I talked about it. I was still attending the adult day care center's support group meetings, so I raised the issue there. "Trust yourselves to know when the time is right to take him out," they advised. There was that answer again, "*You'll* know when the time is right."

As with some things in life, it pays to be patient. The *right* time came three months after he was admitted. (During this period, David and I had been to Milwaukee.)

∽

We didn't know what to expect when we brought Mardig home for a visit. How would he feel? What mood would he be in? Did he have enough sleep the night before? How would he behave once we brought him home? Would Mardig refuse to return to the facility?

I phoned the facility in advance and told the charge nurse our plans. I asked if she would help us by making sure Mardig was dressed and shaved before our arrival. This way, he'd know he was going out.

We arrived with cheerful optimism and tried to hide our underlying awkwardness. When we saw Mardig, he was clean-shaven and dressed. He refused to wear a dress shirt, preferring a T-shirt; cream-colored pleated cotton pants, with the pant legs tucked into his heavy, white athletic socks; and black leather Velcro-fastened athletic shoes.

With great enthusiasm and big smiles we asked Mardig if he wanted to see a movie. His response paled next to our high energy. We had videotaped each of the rooms in his home and my sister and brother while we were in Milwaukee. Mardig looked puzzled, so we explained again and asked if he wanted to see what we had to show him.

He didn't answer our question. Instead he asked if we would bring him back home. We replied, "Of course, we'll bring you back!"

He jokingly replied, "Then I'll go . . . can't get a better deal than that!"

David retrieved a boldly striped cotton shirt from Mardig's closet. Mardig put it on but refused to tuck it into his pants. *This was a change for a man concerned about how he looked.* Either way, we just wanted to take him out. We were ready to leave when he asked, "How do I look?"

"Just great! Only one more thing, please brush your teeth." I was debating whether to ask him to brush his teeth and decided it would be better if he did. I wanted to enjoy his company. I wanted to feel free to lean close to him and speak in his ear when he couldn't hear. I didn't want to have to hold my breath because his was unbearable.

"Is my breath really bad?" Mardig was forthright about such things when he perceived someone cared.

"Yes," I nodded.

"Okay."

I pulled out his grooming kit, handed him the toothbrush, and put a little dab of toothpaste on the brush. He sat on the edge of the bed and began brushing his teeth. Once his mouth started to foam with paste he stood up. Disoriented, he tried to leave the room. I gently directed Mardig to his bathroom, where he continued to thoroughly brush his teeth and gums.

When he finished, I held the toothbrush holder for him so he could slide his brush into it. Confused, he kept placing his hand on the bottom of the container. He feared the toothbrush would slide right through and onto the floor. Once he slid his toothbrush in, I put on the cover. By this time, he was holding onto the entire holder with both hands, unsure what would happen if he let go. I encouraged him to release his hands and then shook the closed toothbrush holder. He smiled, realizing his brush was safely inside.

These are the little things we noticed as he lived each moment with this dementing disease. Alzheimer's is taking its toll. I watch as my father tries harder to make sense of the things most of us take for granted.

We walked out of his room and went to the front desk to sign him out. Then we walked outside. He looked at the busy street in front and asked, "Hey, which street is that?" He wanted to get his bearings.

We got into the car and started driving to our house; about four miles away. He didn't seem as concerned about the streets while in the car. He had lost his new bifocal glasses a few weeks prior, so he couldn't focus on all the previously fascinating things as we drove: street names, tall trees, power lines, and poles. Mardig sat in the front seat next to David. I noticed his breathing was heavy and sometimes he wheezed. "David, I wonder if he caught a cold." I said.

"I wouldn't doubt it."

As we pulled onto the street off the main avenue, Mardig asked, "Is this the street to our home?"

"Yes. Wow, you remember!" After a few more turns, we pulled into our driveway and parked in front of the garage.

"Is this *your* home?"

"Yes."

He got out of the car with a little help and walked up the driveway to the front walkway, which was partially flooded from the lawn sprinklers. He carefully tried to walk around the water puddles, and then dried his feet on the doormat.

Once inside, he looked around. "Hey, is this *your* home?"

"Yes."

"Have I been here?"

"Yes, Mardig. You lived here for six months. Here, have a seat." David directed him to the rocking chair we had placed in front of the television set. We began by showing him pictures of his children and his house in Milwaukee. I pulled out the video camera to capture this moment.

"Mardig, do you know who this is?" David asked, pointing at my picture.

"No," he said hesitatingly.

"How about this one?" David showed him my brother's picture.

"No," he said, his eyes starting to close.

"How about this?" David showed him a picture of his Milwaukee home.

With his eyes still closed, his head dropped onto his chest.

I quickly put down the video camera and ran up to him. *Did he die?* No, he fell asleep.

"Mardig, we have a video to show you of your house in Milwaukee!" I said excitedly.

His eyes opened and he turned his head slightly to look; then his eyes closed again.

We went ahead with our plan to show him the video. Mardig drifted in and out of sleep.

"Mardig, look at this basement," I said, pointing to the television screen that showed the cluttered basement where he had spent a lot of time.

"It was cleaner when I left it," he said tiredly. Then he sat up, "Wow, I wish I had all those tools!"

He struggled to stay awake. We guessed he might have stayed awake the night before. Only an hour had passed when panic overcame him.

"I don't want to die! I don't want to die here! I must go home now. Take me home! I must go home now." He got up and walked toward the front door.

Disappointed and surprised, we turned off the television set, quickly put on our shoes, walked out to the car, and took him *home*.

Once we pulled into the parking lot, he asked, "Is this home?"

"Yes," we said. After he followed us up the ramp, through the entrance and the lobby, and finally into the section where he recognized the other residents, his concerned frown relaxed into a smile. He walked toward his room. We followed him. Without a word, he took off his shirt and pants. Assuming he was getting ready for bed, I pulled back the covers. "Thank you," he said and climbed in bed. David helped pull the covers over him. Mardig then asked us to turn off the lights as we left.

What was that all about? Our home is no longer *his* home. His home is the skilled nursing facility. Perhaps this was a good thing. At first, he tried to get out. Now, he felt safe because it was home. Still, it was unnerving for David and me to know Mardig would much rather go to a relatively sterile room with a single bed and two roommates, instead of being comforted in our home. Perhaps we should be thankful he was happy living there and accept that we had made the right decision.

CHAPTER 15

The Estate Sale

I returned to Milwaukee a month later. I was energized by the fun I had with my siblings in April and their promises to help, so I anxiously phoned them. While waiting for their return calls, Mardig's infinite piles of papers beckoned me. David and I had mailed and carried some of his important papers to California, in order to process them during free moments, but *there was still too much to go through!*

There was more *stuff*, regardless of where I looked. Even though my brother had moved out since my last visit, our earlier efforts hardly made a dent! There were still boxes in the living room. I looked in two of them and found paperwork that seemed to be my brother's. Relieved at not having to process more papers, I moved these boxes into the dining room. (My brother had claimed the dining room as his home office after we stopped using it for meals during my early teens.) But something told me to check these boxes again. I looked inside, paged through some of the papers, and found Mardig's records among my brother's papers. They had to be sorted.

Feeling frustrated and hoping my brother would look though his own papers, I called him. His office manager said he was unavailable. I left a message with her. "This is Brenda, his sister. I'm back in town and need his help. There are boxes with his paperwork mixed with our father's. We need to finish getting through our parents' things. Please tell him to call me as soon as possible so we can get this finished." I hung up the telephone and faced reality. *There were all those boxes upstairs we didn't get to in April! What have I done? Why aren't they here? I'm alone! I can't do this by myself!* Tears filled my eyes. I couldn't cry. I tried to be strong. I needed help.

Could I just turn my back on this? Here I was, my father's POA. What if I threw everything away, and there were valuables, like his savings bonds or cash? Would I be held responsible? Who would know? I didn't plan for all of this! David and I just wanted to help care for Mardig. Managing his affairs was killing me! Maybe, if I stuck with it, I'd grow from the experience. I would learn things. Only those who suffer real hardship can really grow in life.

I tried to see the positive side. Yet, increasing frustration clouded my rosy picture.

I hate this! Why did I have to do all this? Why wasn't my brother helping me? After all, he'd lived in the house for forty-five years rent-free! What kind of person uses his parents without helping them? He never called when Mardig came to California. Mardig left Milwaukee in September, and by January, I asked my sister again, "Have you heard from [our brother]?" "No." "Have you?" "No." What was I doing here, taking care of all this when I was the youngest child and the first to leave the house? Why didn't my parents take care of all this stuff?

I hated my parents' irresponsibility, procrastination, and their greed to accumulate so much. Why wasn't my sister here? I should just throw all this away. To hell with them! They don't care. My father never took the initiative to arrange his matters. After all, didn't I do what I set out to do? I brought him to California to care for him, because I knew he would not survive the Wisconsin winter.

I stood among my parents' possessions . . . all the things they kept from me because they didn't want me to know what they had. And here I was, taking care of it all.

At the depth of my loneliness and self-pity I received a surprise. My brother's girlfriend, whose family just went through a similar cleaning out process after her mother died, empathized. She offered to help. She cared a lot for my brother and thought helping might allow her to learn more about his family. There was only one minor inconvenience; she did not have a car. I offered to drive her, but she preferred to have my brother bring her to the house. They had recently moved fifteen miles away from Mardig's house.

While she was with me, she worked hard and proved to be invaluable. I couldn't thank her enough. She felt embarrassed every time I said thank you. She didn't think it was necessary. She was a kind and caring person. She gave me insight to the human side of my brother, a side of him I forgot after we had grown apart. It was with her I sat in the master bedroom and finished going through my mother's things. It was with her I shared memories of my childhood.

Sharing these memories with my sister and brother would have been much nicer. I would have liked to hear more of their recollections of our childhood, just like they shared in April. But neither of them came this time.

Where were they? Why weren't they returning my calls? They knew I would be here.

My brother made promises he rarely kept. He'd say he'd come to the house for an evening meeting but wouldn't show. He didn't even phone. My sister and I had to reschedule. He promised to support me with the legal issues. Instead, he *erected* legal hurdles for me to navigate. He promised to pick up his girlfriend at a given time. He came much later than promised or not at all.

Despite my pleas, his girlfriend repeatedly declined my offers to drive her home. My brother said his home address and phone number were none of my business. I didn't want to pressure his girlfriend in this awkward situation, especially since she deferred to him. I was grateful for her help and that my brother *allowed* it.

One evening, when he didn't come or phone, she asked if she could spend the night. During the years they were together, she said she had never been in the house alone. She wanted to see what it was like to spend a night in Mardig's house by herself. There was no phone, no food, and none of the comforts of home. I didn't see any harm in it, so we looked for some clothes for her to change into, since she had not come prepared. She didn't mind roughing it for one night.

When I confronted my brother about his lies, he gave one excuse after another about how busy he was—just like our sister. Years earlier, immediately after our mother died, I remember calling him for advice on the style of urn he thought our mother would like. He and our mother had a close relationship; yet, I could not understand why neither he nor my sister chose to be involved when we tried to plan a family memorial service. His advice, "You take care of it. I trust you. I'm busy."

I grew tired of their excuses. *I gave up my career to handle this for the past eight months! Mardig's affairs occupied over one hundred hours of David's and my time in April. We averaged fifteen hours per day. Some days we only had six hours to shower, eat, sleep, and take care of our personal needs. Despite our long hours, here I was again. I was only asking them for ONE week!*

For five days, I averaged twelve-hours a day. My brother's girl-friend helped during much of that time. We were trying to get things ready for the estate sale. When my sister wouldn't answer her phone or call me back, I sent her e-mails instead. At least she might *read* my words. I also journaled my experiences and feelings in e-mails I sent to David. One afternoon, I called my aunt and uncle. They reminded me why I was doing all of this. Both talked into the speakerphone, "Marty was a nice man." "You're doing good things for him. I know he really appreciates it." "Your father used to read a lot . . . in fact, he wouldn't go out. He'd stay in his room and read." "It's sad he had to get Alzheimer's." "He is a good man," my uncle summarized, before asking the question he repeatedly asks when we talk about my taking care of Mardig's affairs: "Have you heard from your sister or brother?"

"No."

"I need to call them . . . find out what's wrong."

"Please do," I'd say with a little self-pity. "I've tried and even sent them e-mails but I haven't heard from them."

"I'll call them. They need to help you. You can't do this all alone."

His words gave me strength.

Since my brother was no longer helping and there was much more stuff to be disposed of, I called the Milwaukee County Department of Public Works and arranged for a trash pickup. After paying nearly $800 for the industrial-sized garbage containers, I learned that because my father owned the house and paid property taxes, the county would pick up the trash for free. One day a crew arrived and together we cleared out the accumulated debris in the backyard.

Without the support of my immediate family I grew adept at creating a family with whomever I could, especially during difficult times. This meant sharing family experiences with others. We had been a very private family. During grade school, we were forbidden to tell our friends what our father did for a living. I never understood why. *What's wrong with telling my classmates my father was a machinist at General Electric X-Ray?* My mother drummed it into our heads. "Our business is none of anyone's business. If someone asks say, 'I don't know.'"

But during this week in May, I reached out to my father's brother. This was important to me, since I did not know Mardig's side of the family very well. Misunderstandings among family members kept us apart throughout much of my childhood. Now an adult, I wanted to judge for myself. I wanted to set these hurts aside and get to know my relatives better. My uncle has Parkinson's disease and is legally blind. He cannot walk very well and needs a wheelchair. We talked frequently by telephone and they invited me to stay with them in their beautiful home in Lake Forest, Illinois. Feeling alone and hopeless one day when my brother did not drop off his girlfriend, I accepted their invitation. I packed an overnight bag and headed south to their home.

I arrived to a delicious home-cooked meal, followed by stories about my father and uncle's upbringing. I looked at my uncle's collection of childhood pictures, including many I'd never seen before.

Then he told me where I could find a large envelope of letters my father had written to him when he served with the Marines during World War II. My uncle saved every letter and returned with them after the war. I stayed up late and read each one. I was struck with awe. (Later, my uncle surprised me by sending a set of copies. What a treasure!)

That night, after stuffing myself with a homemade meal, reminiscing, and getting to know my family, I was ready to be adopted by two caring relatives. I slept on a king-sized bed in one of their bedroom suites, complete with private bathroom, walk-in closet, phone, and television. *This was better than a fine hotel! I didn't want to leave.*

The following morning, I whined about having to face all the work that remained. Although they couldn't help with the physical labor, they offered to visit during the estate sale. That was all I needed to hear and I returned to my father's house with renewed energy.

My brother's girlfriend returned. She apologized for not being able to join me the day before. I told her it was fine because I also needed a break. Unfortunately, she didn't get a break. My brother needed her to get some urgent work finished.

While we cleaned, we shared family stories. I appreciated her kindness, understanding, empathy, and genuine interest. When I became overwhelmed preparing my parents' things for the upcoming estate sale, she'd encourage me to continue. Her interest, assistance, and words helped me approach the end of my major responsibilities in Milwaukee as Mardig's POA. She was a comforting family substitute during my stay in Milwaukee.

The cleaning crew I hired arrived and accomplished what should have been done thirty years earlier—a complete cleaning of the house. The windows, the wall sconces, chandeliers, furnishings, built-in bookshelves, and oriental rugs, *everything*! When they were finished, *I wanted to move in!*

∞

The day before the sale, the estate administrator and her crew helped us with eleventh-hour preparations. Her crew carried boxes outside from the basement and filled the entire backyard! She made sure everything was arranged in an attractive fashion inside the house, from the attic down to the basement.

She encouraged me not to attend the estate sale. She said family members find it difficult to see people place monetary value (usually low) on their family treasures and oftentimes interfere, resulting in her losing a sale. I thanked her for warning me, but insisted on being present. I promised her, if I could not bear to see our treasures leave in strangers' hands, I would leave. Besides, I wanted to experience the process since I had never been through it before. And there was a feeling I had about her and the crew she had assembled from a troubled youth center. I can't explain why, but I didn't trust them. It might have been my uncertainty about the whole experience.

She tried to impress me with the stature of her previous clients, but I was only interested in one thing—selling everything at the highest price. She offered to try to sell Mardig's house during the estate sale. She said sometimes people come through and are more interested in the house than the things inside. I told her if she could sell it for the appraised value or more, she should do it and I would give her a finder's fee.

Our plan was to meet early the next morning before the sale began to do some last minute coordinating.

My brother told his girlfriend to inform me he would be at the estate sale at 1:00 p.m. to help.

The estate sale was about to begin. I wanted to capture everything on videotape beforehand. The estate sale administrator's assistant agreed to videotape me while I walked around and described everything. We started outside on the sidewalk. A wide-angle shot included the house with me standing in the foreground. Just as I began saying a few words about the house and the park across the street, a van pulled up. In a matter of seconds, the passenger door opened and a little black dog ran out. A woman followed, chasing after and shouting at the dog running down the sidewalk. We stopped taping. She scooped up the dog and scolded it as she carried it back to the van. Then she returned and took one look at me.

The childhood bully immediately came to mind. "No, it can't be!" I said to myself.

When I was in fifth grade, the class bully would approach me on the playground and taunt me. I'd try to ignore her, but she'd hit me. I'd walk away, but she and a group of girls would follow. This happened repeatedly. One time, I couldn't take it anymore. She hit me hard, and I began to cry. I was afraid and embarrassed.

As the years passed, she'd come into my mind, and I'd wonder, What happened to her? Is she a successful professional somewhere? Did she drop out of school? Did she have children? Where does she live?

"I went to school with your sister . . . or, maybe, you! What's your name?" she demanded.

I shuddered. *The bully's back!* "Brenda," I promptly replied. *It is twenty-seven years later, and I am still conditioned to reply immediately.*

Before I could think of how to ask my question, she spit out, "How old are you?"

"Thirty-seven."

"Then I went to school with *you*!"

Uh-ohhh, could this be? Nahhh, no way! I try to keep my composure and all the while want to doubt my instinct. I reply, as nonchalantly as I can, "Oh, really . . . and what's your name?" *Please don't say it. Pleeeeassseee!*

She says her name. *It's her! I can't believe it! Can it be the same bully who beat up on me at Hayes Elementary School and actually made me cry? No, please let it not be her.* After twenty-seven years, could it really be her? Once again, I struggle to control my emotions. I say her name, pause, and then repeat it. I feign thought . . . "Are you the [her name] who used to beat up on me at Hayes?"

"Yes, I am," she replied sheepishly.

"Wow!" *What else could I say?*

She explained something about a lack of proper upbringing and beating up others as a way to cope. *Yeah, beating up on ME!* I stopped listening for a moment. "I'm sorry," she said. "I have changed." *I should hope so! She has her own children now.*

"Wow!" I said again. *I couldn't think of anything else to say. After all these years, I was face-to-face with the bully, at my father's estate sale.*

Despite our history, I tried to be nice to her while she looked at items to buy in the house. In fact, as she walked around, I introduced her to a few other people as the girl who used to beat up on me in grade school. Embarrassed, she tried to silence me by furrowing her brows and shaking her head while she placed an index finger over her lips. *With newly gained confidence, from her weakness, I continued flaunting the truth.*

Ironically, I was thrilled and thankful she introduced herself. I was able to close this chapter of my life. I avoided many years of therapy in a few brief minutes during my father's estate sale.

Our meeting had a funny ending. She approached the estate sale administrator with her purchases. I introduced her to the administrator as a person with whom I had went to grade school. This was all I said. The administrator looked at the items and totaled what she owed. After she paid and departed, the people I had told the truth to earlier, and who were waiting to pay for their items, asked if I tried to pull her hair or kick her out of the house. The administrator was puzzled. They explained that she used to beat up on me. The administrator looked at me and exclaimed, "I didn't know she used to bully you. I gave her a discount!"

The estate sale was physically tiring and, much to my surprise, emotionally draining as well. Seeing my parents' things go out the door in strangers' hands was difficult. "What did they pay for that?" I asked the estate sale administrator repeatedly. The prices didn't make sense. Things that should have sold inexpensively captured higher prices. Things that deserved higher prices sold for a low price. And then there was the issue of the administrator herself.

I had not slept much the night before and was up by 5:00 a.m. I was tired. All of my energy was spent. It was already after one o'clock and I had not yet eaten. *I guess my brother would not keep his promise.*

My aunt and uncle arrived. What a joyful sight! I had allies! Seeing I was exhausted, they suggested I get away for a while to eat lunch. I didn't want to at first, but at their insistence, I asked my brother's girlfriend to keep her eye on things while I took a brief break. She assured me she would. I promised to return with lunch for her.

When I returned to Mardig's house, I was surprised to see my sister. She looked equally surprised to see our aunt and uncle. We sat in their Chevy Suburban for a while and talked. Then my aunt went inside to see what was for sale and came out with a hammer. Before leaving, she asked if she could dig up two maple saplings to plant at her home in honor of my father. I was touched by her request and said, "Yes." Later they left, and my sister stayed.

She started asking a lot of questions about the estate sale. She made highly critical comments, telling me how things should be done and for what they should sell. She even challenged the estate sale administrator, who later told me she was offended by my sister's remarks. Despite my concerns about the administrator, I had warned her about my sister and brother's potential reactions.

I was not in the mood to listen to my sister's *after-all-the-hard-work-was-done* criticism. We began to argue. I was tired and lost patience with her. I told her, "You are selfish and self-centered. You never thought about all the tasks I had to accomplish with Mardig's house. You only think narrowly about your own life. You never contemplated the ludicrousness of a person traveling two thousand miles to take care of something a person who lives only five blocks away could handle." She walked out the door, got into her car, and did not speak to me again.

I was fuming. I told my brother's girlfriend, "If she were my daughter . . ."

She finished my sentence, ". . . you'd put her in a convent!" We laughed.

The estate sale was over. A lot remained. People showed up offering cents on the dollar. I couldn't bear them taking advantage of us and turned them away.

My brother still had not come for his girlfriend and we were tired and hungry. We left Mardig's house at 6:30 p.m. and went to David's brother's house to make a few phone calls.

She called my brother's pager and left a message with his answering service. They promised to contact him immediately. We waited and waited. Our disappointment was wearing on us. We sipped beers to offset our hunger and dampen our anger (mostly mine). At 9:45 p.m., after enduring constant stomach growls and feeling shaky from lack of food, I suggested we have dinner. We decided on a Greek restaurant near her home. It was shortly before midnight and after she agreed, I took her home. I had a hard time keeping my eyes open on the way back to my in-laws, where I had been spending the nights during this trip.

Days later, the unsold items were donated, the house was sold for more than the appraised value, the contents sold for half of what the estate sale administrator estimated, and I was left with a few regrets. I knew in my heart if my sister and brother were involved from the beginning, we would have done better for our father and ourselves. Sure, we would have quarreled. We're siblings. But if we went through it, we would have shared memories and become stronger as a family. Plus, we might have kept more of our family treasures, including the Persian rugs my parents had for many years. But there was the fear of one of us retaliating against the other for unequal division of property. So, nearly everything was sold, given away, or dumped.

After I returned to California, another detail remained unresolved. The estate sale administrator wanted her fee for finding a buyer for the house. Since the sale had not yet closed, I could not justify sending her a fee. I explained this to her and she kept insisting as we debated the definition of "finder."

Concerned whether I was being fair, I called the real estate agent in Milwaukee who helped me earlier. She informed me only those who held a real estate license could legally collect fees for *selling* or *finding* a buyer for a house. The estate sale administrator did not have such a license. *Theoretically, I did not have to pay her, given the real estate agent's advice. But a deal is a deal and I would hold up my end of the bargain. Besides, with the competitive bids during the auction, it sold for more than I expected.*

I told the administrator I would send her the fee *after* the sale was final. She was not satisfied, but what could she do?

In contrast, she never sent me a *signed* copy of her appraisal per our agreement.

These annoying details made me appreciate this experience was now behind me.

After all I'd been through during the last eight months, I expected the worst was over. No more fifteen- to eighteen-hour days trying to do a job I later learned takes months. From now on, I could *enjoy* visits to Milwaukee. In California, only small details remained. I would easily fit them into my schedule. I could take care of *my* businesses, which had suffered due to my neglect.

CHAPTER 16

Sexuality Under the Influence of Dementia

Mardig was the ideal diplomat, a perfect gentleman. Even though he spent some of his teen years on the streets of Chicago, he emerged a polite and respectful adult. He always told me to be polite and to treat people with respect, especially those in authority

"Mr. Avadian is engaging in sexually inappropriate behavior."

What exactly does this mean?

Many years earlier, a few of my childhood friends asked if I knew any naughty words in Armenian. I repeatedly asked Mardig, and he denied knowing any. David once asked if I knew any sexual jokes in Armenian. I returned to my father and pleaded, "C'mon, Mardig, tell me a dirty joke in Armenian." He said he didn't know any. I don't recall my father telling a sexual joke in English either. I viewed him as discreet and proper regarding sexual matters.

So, I was taken by surprise at the June quarterly care plan review meeting when the department representatives seated around the table revealed Mardig's behaviors to me.

As with the first meeting three months earlier, I immediately sense an adversarial tone. Instead of an attitude of, *How can we work to-gether for the common good?* this session felt like, *We'll give you this information, and we urge you to do what we say.* Now, it could be due to the dramatic way my father established his reputation on the first day when he disappeared only to be found wandering in the Mojave Desert. Or it could be his going into others' rooms, rummaging through their things, misplacing his hearing aid, and sometimes being uncooperative during his showers. I know he can be a handful.

Still, this is a 200-bed specialized Alzheimer's facility. The staff should know how to deal with these kinds of behaviors. Heeding my father's advice about treating others with respect, I was determined to work with the staff, whose livelihoods involved taking care of my father. I aimed for a healthy exchange of ideas.

When I didn't agree with them, they perceived me as being difficult. When I gave them feedback, I got the impression they'd take it out on Mardig.

My requests were reasonable. "My father's glasses are still missing. Can you please find them?" "My father's gums are getting infected and his front top teeth are looking grayer. Are you making sure the aide brushes them at least once a day?" Yet, I feared they would find little ways to make life difficult for Mardig, or worse, remove him from the facility for a *legitimate* reason. I learned of two instances where residents were removed and the families had little recourse.

On the other hand, if I were afraid to give feedback, what would happen? My father might not be cared for the way he deserved. "It shouldn't be this difficult," I kept telling myself. But it was. I don't know how to proceed. For $120 per day—nearly $44,000 per year—in a three-person room, my father should be cared for just a little more.

"Mr. Avadian has not changed much," the nurse says.

This catches me off guard because I've noticed a big change in his ability to recall who I am. He doesn't realize I am his daughter. Sometimes I am his son. Most of the time, I am a familiar face, making him feel comfortable and safe, a person who will rescue him from his perceived troubles. On rare occasions, I am one of his parents, his Ma or Pa; gender doesn't make a difference.

"What do you mean, 'He hasn't changed much'?"

The social services representative explains. "Mr. Avadian continues to wander, and he even got out of the facility a couple of times
when visitors were leaving."

*Didn't we cover this subject—in detail—with the administrator and
director of nurses when Mardig first escaped? We were told many residents
pose this problem to varying degrees, especially during the first few days.
Given the potential serious consequences, I decide to offer some common-
sense suggestions once more.*

"We covered this in detail six months ago when my father was
wandering in the Mojave Desert. It could have been worse. He could
have frozen to death. Fortunately, he was found and he was unharmed." *I hear the dietician's sigh of relief.* "I suggest the staff monitor
the doors closely and urge visitors to be careful when they leave."

Strangely, they appear unconcerned while I'm speaking. They
barely make eye contact, and look through their notes or elsewhere
in the room. I stand to demonstrate how we can open and then close
the door behind us to make sure no one slips through. I think this
demonstration is common sense, therefore unnecessary; but I proceed, because Mardig's life depends on it. One of the committee
members is not even watching. No one is taking notes. *Of course not!
Why should they? This is common sense!* "You should post a sign asking
visitors to be sure to close the door behind them as they leave, so residents cannot leave accidentally." I demonstrate how I look behind
me as I pull the door closed to make sure it is latched.

*I am convinced my words and demonstrations are falling upon deaf
ears and blind eyes, so I sit down.*

"Mr. Avadian no longer asks for pencils, pens, maps, or phone
books."

*My father used to take notes and look up banks and people's names he
remembered in the phone book. He was an avid note taker and kept
detailed journals. After he lost his glasses, his desire to read and write
waned.*

"Mr. Avadian still walks around *on a mission*. He resists our
attempts to redirect him."

I try to offer one more unsolicited suggestion despite their lack of attention to my last one. "You need to be patient. Try to connect with my father before trying to redirect him." *Only the walls are listening.*

With no acknowledgement to what I've said, the social services representative speaks: "Mr. Avadian organizes other people's drawers. He is up all night wandering, setting off alarms when he tries to exit a door, and disturbs residents during sleeping hours by rummaging through their drawers." *Wow, I remember how it was when he lived with us. We could not sleep the whole night uninterrupted.*

"What else is my father doing?"

The representatives start to fidget and look awkwardly in different directions. The nurse speaks slowly, "Your father relieves himself inappropriately." She pauses for my reaction.

Who comes prepared for this? Toward the end of his stay with David and me, he'd miss the toilet altogether. We'd later find urine on the toilet and down the sides, on the vanity and bathtub, and we'd see puddles on the floor and stains on his clothes. He'd confuse anything white with the toilet. He once pulled down his pants and sat on our French provincial couch in order to have a bowel movement. He even managed to get up onto the washer and was irritated when we tried to stop him. "Can't a person go to the bathroom in peace?" He was able to express himself without being aware of what he was doing.

Wanting to be sure I understood what they meant, I asked, "What do you mean?"

"He relieves himself in the corridors."

"Oh, really?" *I know this is difficult for the staff. This facility is kept clean. In fact, if the powerful smell of cleaning solution is any indication, the place is being cleaned constantly.* "What else does he do?"

This time they look at one another and then the activities coordinator says, "He exposes himself."

He does what? My father? "Really? How so?" I ask as calmly as I can muster.

"Well, we saw him holding himself in the dining room."

"Hmmm." *I try to keep a straight face while fighting off my disbelief.* I paraphrase for clarification, "You mean, he unzips his pants and holds himself?"

"Yes."

"Have you seen him do this?" I ask the social services director who responded so quickly.

"No. I got it off the report." *The nursing staff maintains weekly reports on each resident. In Mardig's case, these reports have become a daily occurrence.*

"Has anyone seen this?" I ask the group in general.

"Yes," the activity representative replies.

"What did he do?"

"Well, he was standing in the dining room holding himself."

"Then what?"

"Well," she hesitated, "he exposed himself to the other residents."

I just couldn't imagine my father doing this.

"What did they do?"

"Oh, some got irritated, others ignored him."

A mischievous and naughty thought popped into my mind: my father can't even be a "turn-on" in an Alzheimer's facility!

"What did you do?"

"Well, I walked in front of him and asked him to put himself away. I told him this behavior was inappropriate."

"Did he understand?"

"Yes, I suppose."

"What did he do?"

"Martin said he couldn't. He smiled sheepishly and said he was hard." *Wow, this is getting embarrassing. My father . . .?*

We are smiling uncomfortably. "So, what did you do?"

"I redirected him away from the other residents and helped him zip his pants."

"Wow." I describe the way my father was and how surprised he'd be if he were aware of what he was doing. This behavior is so foreign to the way he lived his life. He was quite the gentleman.

"This is typical behavior for some of the residents who were sexually proper," the nurse volunteers.

I know this can be normal behavior for some people with Alzheimer's. My father is not aware of what he is doing because the disease is destroying his brain. I cannot fault him. I can only accept what is. I heard other family members say one woman routinely took off her clothes and paraded up and down the halls of the facility. Another man regularly brought women into his room.

"What else does he do?"

Again, they glance at one another, as if to decide if they should tell me.

"He urinated in a cup and then offered it to a female resident."

"Hah, like an offering!" I exclaim, desperately trying to lighten up the heaviness in the room.

The dietary and activities representatives chuckled. The nurse and social services representatives remained serious.

"What else does he do?"

"He tries to bring women into his room."

"Have you seen this?" I ask the social services representative who tells me this.

"No, but I've read the reports and one of the aides said she went into his room and saw him with another woman."

I think it is nice Mardig is trying to enjoy himself. However, given his cognitive state and that of the other residents, I wonder about the risk of physical injury and emotional pain. A very young child catching her parents making love may see the act as painful. I mention this to the committee. They appear to accept these comments graciously.

I think about how awful this would be for the husbands of the female residents. For example, I imagine if Jonathan, who visits his wife frequently, would walk in and see my father with his wife.

Is this like taking care of children? I wonder. I mean, we have to be serious about what our children do. We can't ignore it. If Mardig, who granted me durable powers of attorney for both health care and financial matters, behaves inappropriately, am I responsible?

The nurse advises me to speak with the director of nurses who will urge me to have Mardig seen by a psychiatrist. "A *psychiatrist*? How can a psychiatrist help someone with Alzheimer's?" I ask.

The nurse says, "Your father's mental condition needs to be evaluated, as does his need for possible medications."

My father has Alzheimer's. What is there to be evaluated? Oh, I know!
The psychiatrist will prescribe drugs. This is the beginning of the end.

Mardig was eighty-six years old and took no medications. This was
highly unusual for a person his age. So, I debated having him start
polluting his body. During the last years of my mother's life, her medication had increased to seven pills, four times a day. The chemical
reactions among the pills to help her enlarged heart function played
havoc with her mind.

I raise the medication issue at our weekly Adult Day Care caregiver
support group. Some disagree that prescription drugs are the
beginning of the end. They argue whatever helps my father function
comfortably with this disease is best. "No use in torturing him as he
tries to live day-to-day. Besides, his aggressive behavior may be a risk
to the other residents, and he may have to be removed from the
facility." This last comment strikes terror in my heart. I prefer Mardig
to be close to home where I can see him often.

The worst may not be over.

I'm afraid. If we don't get medications for Mardig, the director of
nurses and her staff could try to make a case for removing him. I
believe they are being too hasty, jumping to a quick solution for a
situation common among people with Alzheimer's. First one pill,
then another, and soon Mardig will become a *zombie!* My mind is
racing. *What should I do? They can't force my father to take drugs. Can*
they?

I call Mardig's doctor and ask his opinion. "I'm concerned about
starting him on any medications," I conclude.

"I understand," he says. "I will be visiting the facility this week and
I'll check on your father." He visits weekly since a significant number
of the residents are his patients. *I wonder if this is why the former*
admissions representative introduced him as their medical director.

"I'd rather not have Mardig take medications unless he absolutely has to." He assures me he will discuss my father's situation with the management.

If he's their medical director, won't he have a conflict of interest? Won't he be inclined to represent the facility's interests rather than Mardig's? On the other hand, if he sees many patients, he'll visit regularly and know more about what happens to people with this disease. Apparently, few doctors regularly visit the facility to check on their patients. This was my dilemma as I waited to hear from him.

I went to the support group for their ideas on handling this doctor's potential conflict of interest. Roberta, who also served as our facilitator, encouraged me to call the doctor and share my concerns.

"You mean my concern with his potential conflict of interest?"

"Yeah, Brenda, why not?"

"Well, because he might get put off by it. I'm on shaky ground with this facility as it is."

"There's nothing wrong with discussing your feelings with your father's doctor. He shouldn't get angry. If he does, you should get another doctor!"

"Well, I'm not sure I want to, considering it is hard to find a doctor to visit the facility."

"Just talk with him, Brenda. You know how to talk with people. He'll understand."

With her encouragement, I called the doctor's office. *I expected he would have called me after seeing Mardig since I had expressed concern.* When I asked if he had seen my father, he said he had. "Well, what do you suggest for him?" Surprisingly, he said the same thing the director of nurses did, "Have a psychiatrist see your father."

I knew it! There is a conflict of interest! My heart beat faster.

"Are there any other options?" I asked.

"You could have Mardig moved to another place where he could receive one-on-one care."

How could he say that? He knows there are no places nearby. Just in case, I want to be sure. "Do you know of any place like that nearby?"

"No."

"Are these my only two options?"

"Yes."

I couldn't think of anything else to say. This wasn't going the way I anticipated. "I'll think about it," I said.

Did the management at the facility talk with the doctor and suggest he strongly recommend Mardig see a psychiatrist, and then be medicated? I did not want to go down this path.

I had to find a way to talk with the doctor face-to-face. It was the only way. The telephone was too awkward.

I had an idea! I still had questions about how I completed Mardig's advance directives according to his wishes when he was admitted. The form gave bipolar choices. Either resuscitate or don't. What if he choked on a chicken bone? He wouldn't want to die. I had written the directive such that Mardig would be resuscitated in the nursing home and then taken to the hospital where doctors could examine him. Depending on their diagnosis, I would follow Mardig's wishes. Mardig did not want to be on life support if the diagnosis was terminal. I heard too many nightmare stories about a loved one being placed on life-support because the doctor or hospital was unaware of a living will. I did not want this to happen to Mardig.

Armed with this approach, I called the doctor's office again and asked to speak with him. When he picked up the telephone, my brain froze. "I'd like to set an appointment to discuss patient philosophy with you." *Oops, that was the wrong thing to say! My abrupt request might imply dissatisfaction with his care. I grew nervous and couldn't think of a way to retract my statement.*

"If you want another physician, it is okay with me," he said.

Wow, I didn't think he would take such offense at my request. I stammered, "I . . . I just want . . . to *talk* with . . . with you."

"We can talk now, on the telephone."

"I would feel better in a face-to-face meeting."

"Why? I'm on the telephone right now. We can talk now."

"I'll feel more comfortable if we're face-to-face. I'll be happy to pay for the doctor's appointment."

"Whatever . . . set an appointment with the receptionist."

"Thank you, I will."

David and I considered if there might be cultural or gender issues affecting my communications with the doctor. David agreed to take time off from work to accompany me to this appointment, just in case the doctor found it difficult to respectfully discuss concerns expressed by a female or by a person challenging a doctor's authority.

We met for forty-five minutes and discussed several issues (medications, desire to stay at the facility, brain activity during comas, and life support). The doctor said he would monitor Mardig's behavior and he urged us to have Mardig seen by a psychiatrist. We agreed to take this route if Mardig's inappropriate sexual behaviors continued. The doctor accepted this. For the moment, David and I finally saw eye-to-eye with the doctor.

Things started looking better. Months passed and Mardig stopped displaying inappropriate sexual behavior. He did not have to be seen by a psychiatrist, and he was not placed on any medication.

Looming overhead was the ever-present issue: *When am I going to get on with my life?* I was exhausted from thinking too much, from tossing and turning during sleepless nights, and from trying to make sense of things about which I knew little. *Why does it have to be like this?*

Caregivers encouraged me with their heartfelt compliments.

"You are such a devoted daughter. Regardless of how you may be getting behind in your life right now, you will be glad you took time to care for your father."

"You won't regret this."

"Your father is so fortunate to have you."

"I wish you were my daughter. When I need care, I wish you would be there."

FOUR

Memories

CHAPTER 17

Finding the Joy

W hen life brings us challenging experiences, we comfort ourselves with that old saying: *We will laugh about this in years to come.* Following are a few of my favorite memories of my father as Alzheimer's took over his life.

MARDIG ATTENDS OUR BUSINESS MEETINGS

When Mardig came to live with us in the fall of 1996, it was a season filled with many social opportunities for him. I enjoyed seeing him smile and laugh with my friends and business partners. In stark contrast to the hermit existence he had adopted in Milwaukee, when he lived with us he showered every other day and was nicely dressed. We even took his clothes to the cleaners. Mardig would comment on the creases in his pants. He looked sharp, he was polite, and people enjoyed spending time with him. After all, he was the consummate gentleman.

Because he wandered, we had to keep him within sight. During weekends and weeknights when we held meetings for our growing television network business, David and I took turns staying home with Mardig. However, over the weeks, this was limiting our progress building the business. Both of us needed to be present at the meetings, and so, with great trepidation, we brought Mardig along one evening. *How many people bring their parent to a business meeting, much less one who has Alzheimer's and occasionally says and does embarrassing things?*

Our fears were unfounded. Our business partners enjoyed him; showering him with lots of attention. Mardig provided enough distraction to counteract the seriousness of our intense planning sessions. He even admitted being *spoiled* by all the attention. Our partners wanted Mardig to return to future meetings.

A petite young lady with long black hair and Mardig smiled and laughed at each other's jokes during one meeting. She even gave him back and shoulder massages. Before another meeting, she invited Mardig to the swing set in the backyard of our host's home. As I watched them swing like children, smiling and giggling, I wished I had my video camera.

MIRROR, MIRROR ON THE WALL

One Sunday afternoon, shortly after Mardig moved into our home, David and I were quietly sitting in the family room reading the mail that had accumulated during the week, when we heard someone talking. Since only the three of us lived in the house, we got up to investigate.

As David and I approached Mardig's room, we heard his voice. We walked to the doorway and peered inside, trying not to be noticed. He was facing the full-length mirrored closet doors, with his hands clasped behind his back, speaking clearly in Armenian, *"Ah-sor maseen, eench guh khor-rees?" Ahsonts guh-nank ohk-nyl?"* ("What do you think about this? Can we help these people?") He waited for a reply. None came, so he repeated the questions. Again, he waited.

David and I looked at each other and then giggled softly, wondering if what we saw was real.

Mardig grew irritated at the unresponsive image. Trying to stand straighter, despite his curved spine due to osteoporosis, he asked, *"Aboosh es? Mee-yan hon guh-gehnas!"* ("Are you dumb? You're just standing there!")

We could barely contain ourselves when we realized he was serious. We didn't know whether to laugh or to cry. Mardig was having a conversation with his reflection!

We returned to the living room and tried to make sense out of what we just saw. This was so different from our everyday experiences; we didn't know what to do.

This behavior continued over the weeks. Mardig would call us into his bedroom and show us the person who was mimicking him. He'd express how irritating it was. Again, we didn't know what to think. He'd say, "Look at him! All he does is mimic me and doesn't answer my questions. He looks stupid." *To think he was speaking of himself— his reflection.*

We tried a few things, including using a video camera to help Mardig understand the difference between his physical self and his image reflected by a mirror or on the television screen. While I held the video camera, David touched Mardig's knee and asked him whose hand was on his knee.

"Yours."

"Who am I?"

"You . . . David."

"Okay, now look at the TV. Who do you see?"

"You!" Mardig exclaimed with a nervous laugh.

"Who's that guy next to me?"

"Well, that's just it. You need to call the station manager. There's a guy that looks just like me on TV! Write a letter to him. I'm serious. That guy looks just like me. They can research it."

"Mardig, who's touching you?"

"You are," my father said, directing his attention to David.

"Look at the TV. Who is touching you?"

"Look, you're there! You're on TV."

"Yes, and who's that man next to me?"

"That guy!"

We went back and forth like this for ten minutes. Mardig couldn't make the leap to understand. He recognized David and me on TV and in person, but he couldn't comprehend his own image on TV or his reflection in the mirror.

Several weeks passed before David came up with the brilliant idea of reversing the closet doors so the mirrored sides faced in. He even got Mardig to help him re-install them one weekend. Despite the closet door frames detracting from the room's decor, this new arrangement certainly gave my father peace of mind.

MARDIG FLIES TO CATALINA ISLAND

My father had been at the skilled nursing facility for about seven weeks when a unique opportunity arose. In March 1997, our good friend Lew was planning a trip to Catalina Island. A superb still photographer, he wanted to visit the island to take pictures. Lew and Mardig got along marvelously. Mardig couldn't explain why he felt so comfortable with Lew, since he'd only met him a few months ago. Nevertheless, David and I knew this would be a fine opportunity for the two buddies to have a fun adventure. (A year earlier David and I had flown to Catalina Island and thought Mardig would also enjoy the trip.)

We had previously scheduled commitments and could not join them. I asked Lew if he'd like to go to Catalina with my father. At sixty, Lew's age misrepresented his youthful vigor. Before he replied, I threw in an incentive. The ferry would take an hour to reach the island from San Pedro. If Lew agreed to take Mardig, we would pick up the tab for the entire day, including the fifteen-minute helicopter flight to and from the island.

Lew accepted.

We arranged with the nursing facility to have Mardig dressed and ready at 5:00 a.m. We wrote a letter granting Lew authority to care for my father and to make any decisions for him should the need arise. We also gave Lew Mardig's identification, a cell phone, and our video camera.

We agreed to meet Lew at the skilled nursing facility at 4:30 a.m. When David and I arrived, we were surprised to see Mardig fully dressed and ready to go. We signed him out, and he accompanied us outside. A palette of orange, pink, and brown strokes previewed the March sunrise. Lew took a few pictures of my father and us with this colorful backdrop. We exchanged hugs and wished both of them well.

David and I watched as Lew and Mardig drove away. It was like seeing our child leaving for summer camp. We were a little nervous because we didn't know what to expect. We hoped for the best. Lew and Mardig would drive down to the port in Long Beach to board a helicopter—my father's first flight in one.

Days later, Lew wrote a detailed diary of their journey and gave us a duplicate set of the pictures he took featuring my father at the Catalina Casino, the Wrigley Museum and grounds, and during the glass-bottom boat tour. He also gave us a photo album and colorful stationery of seashells and images of the sea. Afterward we assembled a beautiful keepsake of my father's excursion to Catalina Island.

MARDIG BOLDY BREAKS THE LAW

One April day, Lew, Mardig, and I went to the California Poppy Preserve in the Antelope Valley. The orange-colored poppy is California's state flower and the preserve is reputed as one of the finest places to see poppy blooms painting hillsides a vivid orange. People come from around the world to see and photograph them each year.

We've been told it is against the law to pick these poppies. So, when we walked among the flowers and Mardig bent down and plucked one out of the ground, we gasped and looked around. Other visitors didn't seem to notice. He carried his victorious acquisition between his teeth with pride. When Lew saw Mardig, he began to laugh. We took plenty of pictures and videotaped him enjoying the windy day as the flowers swayed from side to side. Fortunately, the Poppy Police did not arrest him.

THERE ARE NO GOOD-BYES—ONLY HELLOS

Good-byes are difficult. When you care about someone, you wish there were no farewells. Lovers struggle to say good-bye when trying to end their telephone conversations. "No, you say it!"

"No, you say it and then we'll hang up."

"I don't want to say 'good-bye.'"

"Okay, we won't say it."

It's the same when your loved one has Alzheimer's. David and I learned there are no good-byes, only hellos. Each time we visit Mardig, we greet him with a hearty hello.

He furls his brow, looks at our faces, and then gives us a big smile. "Boy, am I glad to see both of you!"

After we've spent an hour or two with him and must leave, we usually just walk away. Sometimes Mardig says, "You're free to stay here and do what you want. I need to . . ." then he walks away, or sits down to rest. Whatever he does, we watch him for a while. When he enters the world he creates in his mind, we see he has forgotten us and we depart.

At first it seemed cruel to just walk away from him. But he really doesn't remember. When we say good-bye it is more painful for him.

"When am I going to see you again?" he asks. Or "Where are you going? I'll come with you."

We've learned if we simply let him be, there's no need to say good-bye.

We realize that one day he will no longer be with us. So, we treasure each moment and focus on hello.

TWENTY-FOUR-HOUR PIZZA DELIVERY

Once Mardig started living in the skilled nursing facility, David and I gave boxes of chocolates or home-baked treats like chocolate chip cookies or *pakhlava* (Armenian flaky pastry filled with a mixture of finely chopped walnuts and pistachios and flavored with honey and cinnamon) to the staff during the holidays. We'd leave three big boxes with the day shift and ask them to be sure a box was given to each of the two following shifts.

After three years, I wanted to do something special and personal for the staff on all three shifts. Despite my father's initial experience at this facility, the staff that actually interacted with Mardig, really liked him and took good care of him. Two staff members even asked permission to take his photo. One had his picture placed in a charm to wear on her bracelet and the other, in the locket of her necklace. I was honored. I had to do something to show our appreciation.

David and I decided to deliver hot pizzas and cold sodas for each shift within a twenty-four-hour period. We asked the staff what they liked on their pizza and told them not to bring lunch on the day we would deliver the pizzas. Then we begged the local pizza shop to stay open an hour later so we could make the final delivery after midnight.

At 11:05 a.m., we arrived with freshly baked pizzas and icy cold sodas for the morning shift. They were thrilled and couldn't believe we actually went through with our plan. We were surprised they didn't believe us. The second shift was also happy and surprised to receive pizzas right out of the oven. They heard we did this for the first shift but didn't realize we'd be doing it for them too. They were expecting the first shift's leftovers.

After this second pizza delivery, we went home tired, knowing we had to make one more delivery. At midnight, we awoke after an hour nap. David vowed he would never agree to another twenty-four-hour delivery. We called the pizza parlor to confirm our order and our one o'clock pick-up time. The night shift would receive an early lunch delivery because the pizza place could not stay open much longer. When we arrived with the pizzas at 1:20 a.m., we rang the doorbell at the back entrance. There was no answer. I called on my mobile phone. No answer. We began wondering what to do with all the pizzas and sodas when someone finally answered the phone.

By one-thirty the door was opened and David and I walked in with bright smiley faces announcing: "Pizza delivery!" The staff was truly surprised. They had no idea, which was a surprise to us because the morning staff said they left notes for the other two shifts. Nearly everyone had brought their lunches because they said no one had ever done anything like this, especially at this hour. As they placed slices of hot pizza on their plates, they thanked us with tears in their eyes. They said how wonderful it was to meet family members because they rarely do, unless it is an emergency. David and I were deeply touched and had to fight back our own tears. It was a special moment.

The three pizza deliveries took a lot out of us, but our fatigue was insignificant to all the pleasure we derived from the staff's surprised reactions and genuine appreciation.

Today, I'm saying we need to do this again. And much to my surprise, David says he'll join me.

CHAPTER 18

The Little Things
Matter Most

S itting in the activity room one afternoon, with Mardig sleeping
in the chair by my side, I observe the residents and occasionally
glance at the television. I wonder what it would be like to live
in an Alzheimer's skilled nursing facility. Then a question begins to
repeat in my mind: *What is the meaning of life?*

So many of us are driven by our needs, goals, wants, and aspir-
ations. We want to be successful in life. What does this mean? If we
judge what successful means by watching television in the U.S., it
means having enough money to buy a new car every two years, a big
home to redecorate every season, gold jewelry accented with dia-
monds, and new clothes to keep up with the ever-changing fashions.
It means taking a vacation twice a year, attending sporting and
cultural events regularly, eating at the finest restaurants, and a cell
phone for every member of the family.

*Do these things really matter? Do any of these things matter to the
people in this activity room?*

These residents don't own many things. In fact, they rummage
around in each other's rooms, closets, and drawers and share what
they have; including, much to my surprise, each other's clothes,
glasses, dentures, and shoes.

Before my father came to the facility, we took him to the eye doctor to get his prescription updated. We bought him an expensive pair of eyeglasses with lightweight plastic lenses that would not make marks on the bridge of his nose like his heavier glasses did. We added a bright red strap with his name clearly printed on it, to hold his glasses around his neck so he would not lose them.

He lost them. We told the social services representative and she found them. He lost them again. They were found. This went on for two or three months. They said Mardig left his glasses in other resident's rooms and took the glasses he found in those rooms. He had an affinity for women's glasses with large colorful frames. For a two-month period, when we visited him, he'd be wearing a different pair. Actually, women's glasses look nice on him. Unfortunately, his glasses were never found again.

The residents rarely wear jewelry. Most don't carry a wallet or purse, and they have little cash, if any. My father usually has a few dollars in his pocket to keep him happy. Most of the residents wear cotton-polyester blend sweatshirts and pants while they're awake and sometimes even while sleeping. They sleep in beds covered with white cotton-polyester blend sheets, and cotton-weave blankets. They bathe twice a week. They eat three meals a day tailored to their nutritional needs. Occasionally they complain about wanting to go somewhere or needing something.

In the activity room, one woman sits in a wheelchair, crying out and pounding on the tray table. Her face is drawn long and her mouth is wide open as her urgent screams convey great pain. The image of a mother crying out in agony at the loss of her husband or child in a war-torn country comes to my mind. I want to reach out to this woman, to comfort her, yet I am frozen. I fear uncertainty. *What if she needs my attention for a long time and Mardig wakes? Can I tear myself away from her to be with him?*

My father is still napping in the chair. I begin to feel anxious. *Why am I sitting here looking around when I have so much work to do? I should have brought work with me. I'm wasting valuable time sitting here waiting for him to wake up.*

I continue looking around the room. An older overweight man wearing a baseball cap, who usually walks along the hallway near Mardig's room, sits, staring. Whenever I walk near him, I am cautious, as I never knew what to expect. His mouth is slightly open and saliva drips onto his plaid shirt. His eyes are deep and intense, and I fear one day he'll lunge out at me and start screaming.

I turn my head and see Elizabeth. She is carefully reading a magazine. Her head moves down as she scans each page, starting at the top and methodically moving to the bottom before turning the page. She has a look of peace about her. She and her husband, Jonathan, spent most of their lives helping others. They are in their early eighties. Elizabeth was diagnosed with Alzheimer's a few years earlier. It saddens me to see her. She was an author. Her book, *The Living Atoms and You,* addresses the significant role atoms play in our everyday lives physically, spiritually, mentally, and emotionally. Elizabeth was also a teacher. For years, many followed her as a source of knowledge and wisdom.

Why? Why is Elizabeth destined to live the rest of her days with Alzheimer's in this facility? Why is the woman pounding on her tray table? Why is the man living his remaining days drooling and stricken with dementia? Why does my father have to live with this disease?

Overall, they seem content, at peace, and occupied in the worlds they create for themselves. They are children with vivid imaginations in aging bodies. This disease helps them believe they travel to many places. In recent months my father's been to England to fight the war, to Africa to stop the poachers, to Wisconsin where he works, to Illinois where he lives with his mother and goes to school, and to New York to do his banking. Many residents still speak of driving every day. Mardig talks about taking the car to visit Ma who is in the hospital or to take her shopping. Some ride a bus. All see their families at one time or another; especially their parents. This is how they survive.

What is the meaning of life? *Life has meaning when we create special memories with people we care for and who care for us. These are life's real treasures when we have nothing more. I am only thirty-eight. Two years*

*ago, I wasn't even aware of this disease. And yet, I am thankful for what I
have learned so far; especially patience and what matters in life.*

I smile at this realization. After all, we never know if we've lived life
correctly until we're finished. And then it's too late. So, I become an
observer of life.

Since the devastation of the 1994 Northridge earthquake and after
clearing out my parents' home, I have been disposing of things.
Families lost their treasured belongings without any warning after the
6.7 magnitude quake. I ask myself, What is absolutely essential if
there's a major disaster and we have to vacate immediately? I do not
have collectibles because they are too much trouble to keep clean.
Not a day goes by when I don't consider what I no longer need and
can give away. The biggest challenge is finding people who can use
the things I want to give away.

My mind drifts; and then I realize, I am here with my father.

When I visit Mardig, I focus on the present. I remind myself to accept
him as he *is*, not as he was or could be. As the disease progresses and
takes its toll on his brain, this becomes more difficult. It is a challenge
to watch him struggle to make sense of his world. It becomes
increasingly difficult emotionally to listen to Mardig desperately try
to make sense of his surroundings. His vocabulary slowly escapes him
and he struggles to find the words to express himself. I watch him try
to recall his family: his children, his wife, his brothers. His world is
gradually shrinking, and he is left only with little things, his memories
of *mere* incidents from years gone by.

In the hours I've spent with Mardig, I've learned little things matter
most.

Mardig's Eighty-Seventh Birthday

David and I want to bring Mardig home to celebrate his birthday,
but this is impractical. He considers the nursing facility his home, and
he feels uncomfortable when he leaves. We don't understand this,

thinking a change of pace would be nice. *After all, wouldn't he like to go out for a while?*

We arrange to bring the birthday celebration to him. We order a butter-cream frosted marble cake. The sweeter the better. He loves sweets! We have it decorated with confetti, ribbons, his name, and "Happy 87th Birthday!" These days, he does not know how old he is; he thinks he is in his thirties or fifties. We bring noisemakers and a cake knife (actually, a long-serrated bread knife), plastic forks, and paper plates.

We invite people who helped care for him while he was living with us: Sally, Jan, Dave, and Roberta. We invite Jonathan and his wife, Elizabeth, and the staff from the facility. We want an intimate group to celebrate Mardig's achievement: eighty-seven years on this challenging journey called life.

On his birthday (it is mine, too) the gathering is just as I'd envisioned. Mardig is happy and even a bit alarmed at all the fuss for him. We still aren't sure he knew it was his birthday. And for a moment, when he picked up the knife to cut the cake . . .

Mardig cuts a piece off the corner of the cake, a heavily frosted piece. He then carefully balances the sweet morsel on the end of the long knife blade. We watch closely, wanting to grab the knife from his hand, yet frozen with fear we might startle him. *I definitely had to give my father credit. He took great pains to be careful. Still, he did have Alzheimer's.* Carefully balancing the cake on the end of the knife, he slowly turns it toward his mouth. We watch, totally speechless. Then the activity director gasps. Mardig looks up and pulls the knife out of his mouth. He is unharmed. We break out laughing with relief and rush to him with a plastic fork. Then we sing *Happy Birthday* as Mardig continues to eat his cake. He has a big smile, with frosting on the outside of his mouth. He is having fun, and so are we.

What a birthday! Even though it was my birthday too, Mardig stole the show with the knife incident.

MY MOTHER IRONING

I remember my mother spending hours ironing each week. I

remember her standing over the ironing board in the master
bedroom upstairs. I remember warm summer days when she'd iron
downstairs in the living room or in the sunroom. When the weather
was especially nice with a gentle breeze blowing, she would take the
ironing outdoors. She'd iron outside of the sunroom, near the dining
room windows. I would stay inside because I was embarrassed. I
didn't want to be seen by the neighbors. *People are not supposed to iron
outdoors!* Eventually I grew used to watching her and even volunteered to help her carry the clothes and iron outside.

Ma ironed my father's pants, shirts (both dress and work), handkerchiefs, and boxer shorts. She would even iron the linen sheets and
pillowcases.

I'd stand by her in the living room and watch, sometimes trying to
help, but mostly getting in the way. She would place the ironed
clothes on the floor, and I'd play with the neatly arranged pants and
shirts. I'd fold the legs on my father's pants to see what kind of funny
contortions I could create. I'd do the same with the arms of his shirts.
She'd shoo me away, but I'd return.

*I wondered, Would I have to iron so much when I grow up? It takes so
much time! It never ends! I'm not going to do this when I grow up. But,
who will? Maybe I'll hire someone to do it for me.*

Remembering these days, I placed a few of Ma's things from
Milwaukee on the ironing board. I tried to carefully iron these treasures without harming them. I stood in Mardig's former bedroom in
our home and began to iron. I pressed doilies, handkerchiefs, pillowcases, and tablecloths. All of these featured Ma's *tsera khordz*
(embroidery in Armenian). My weak wrist began to ache.

It's been over thirty years since I thought about Ma ironing. Today
I am her and *Little Brenda* is standing by my (*her*) right side. *Brenda is
wearing a wrinkled dress, white anklets with embroidered designs, and
black patent leather shoes. She wants to help.* I stand there quietly, ironing. And then I watch her from Little Brenda's perspective. She
carefully lays out the material and then glides the steaming iron over
it, being careful not to accidentally press a crease into the material or
get the tip of the iron caught in the embroidered designs.

Wow, such work! Such labor-intensive work.

I do not want to spend the weekend ironing. David and I take our clothes to the laundry because it takes us too long to iron one item. Still, I *need* to iron these things. I feel I am honoring my mother. And it is the one time I feel able to understand the extent of her responsibility. She would say, "Wait until you have kids, you'll understand." David and I are in our late thirties and we have not started a family. *Yet at this moment, I think I understand, if only a little.*

In honor of and in my mother's memory, I feel renewed strength. I stand and iron all of the pieces of her *tsera khordz* and then wrap them carefully in tissue paper and place them inside white gift boxes. I will pull them out from time to time and display them on my furniture. I will *use* them. Ma had packed them away. Each time I look at them or a guest comments on them, I will acknowledge my mother's efforts. In this way, her work will be seen and she will be remembered.

SIBLING RIVALRY

There are three of us. My brother is eight years older than me. My sister is the middle child and older than me by two years. The more I think about our upbringing, the more I realize we were raised to be competitive.

If there's anything that fostered healthy competition, it was when we played checkers with Mardig. Occasionally Ma gave us competitive advantage when she sat close enough to Mardig to sneak one of his pieces *off* the checkerboard! She could do this quite easily since he focused intensely on each move and seemed to lack peripheral vision. Most of the time, we'd laugh, because we couldn't believe Mardig actually focused so hard. He would look puzzled, wondering why we were laughing. We'd confess the dirty deed. Ma, having been caught, would look off in another direction with saintly innocence. *Moi?*

Our height was another source of competition. My brother was the tallest, then my sister, and then little ol' me! I still have not won this sibling competition. But I finally grew taller than my father! That was a major coup.

So there I was, wondering what I could win because my older sister and brother were so much better at everything than me. (They made certain I remembered how much better they were, too.)

When I think of it, it's truly amazing how, despite being raised in the same house by the same parents, we're so different. When my friends and I discuss how our upbringings have affected us I realize I could have turned out worse. I could have given up. Or, I could have sought competitive environments where winning was the only thing that mattered in life.

Still, what could I do to win? What was the one thing I could be better at than my sister or brother? Since they are older and had a head start, what was left?

My time came when I graduated from high school at the age of sixteen. By the time I was in my second year of college, I felt constrained living with my parents. I was the rebel, the one who tried new things, the one who went contrary to our parents' wishes. I was an independent, know-it-all eighteen-year-old. I needed to spread my wings. I moved out a few months after my eighteenth birthday. My sister moved out soon after. She was twenty. My brother stayed at home until he was forty-six, shortly before I arranged to sell Mardig's house. *They lost! I won! That's one victory for me!*

I believe I won in other areas as well. Unlike my siblings, without my parents' financial support I earned a college degree and went on to earn a master's degree. It was hard and the money would have been nice, but I learned a lot about survival and succeeding, despite many obstacles and temptations along the way.

Today, I don't have a *need* to *win*. I proved to myself I could set goals and achieve them. I do not need to compare myself to my brother or sister. What is important is accomplishing *my* goals.

What is the Meaning of Life?

Once again, this question runs through my mind. As I wait for my father to wake up, I wonder about the people in this room. *What, in their lives, leaves some with great pain, like the woman pounding on her tray table; others with warm memories; and the rest at peace, like*

Elizabeth? Why do some residents have visitors and others don't? Are these reasonable things to think about?

Do the stereotypical measures of success matter in life? Would people care more for me if I had front-row center seats at the Ahmanson Theater in Los Angeles? Would people care if I dined at five-star restaurants? Does it matter that I drove a convertible along the entire California coastline? Or that I receive annual invitations from Kentucky's governor to attend a barbecue before the Kentucky Derby? Does it matter that some of my investments yield high returns?

Will any of these things matter when I'm pounding my fist on the tray table attached to my chair, scanning each page of an old magazine, drooling on my shirt, or sleeping in a chair in front of the television set in an Alzheimer's facility's activity room?

NO! Who would even know? Who would care?

When life takes nearly everything away from us, the little things will matter most.

CHAPTER 19

A Rare Gift

Mardig is still alive as I write this book. It is a windy fall day and on the car seat next to me are the carefully chosen pages that may hold Mardig's interest. I want him to read at least a portion of this book, even though his comprehension is not what it used to be.

Whenever I accomplish a major feat in life (like writing this book), I think of my parents. I wonder how they would react or what they might say. The older I get, I realize more of my behaviors, thoughts, and values, mirror theirs. Perhaps I desire Mardig's praise or yearn for his warm smile, a compliment, or a pat on the back—the kind only a parent can give.

Mardig no longer makes sense out of most of what he reads. When he derives meaning from something, it becomes his reality. Months earlier he retrieved an old issue of *National Geographic* and read an article about poachers in Africa. He spent the rest of the day thinking he was living in Africa trying to stop the poachers. He'd sometimes invite us to join him on these missions. After reading an article in *Life*, he had to leave immediately for England (his imagined homeland) to fight with his fellow countrymen in World War II. Realizing this, I was prepared to accept whatever his reaction would be, even if it involved his taking the train from California to England during the war!

Mardig is walking in the hallway as I approach. He looks up at me, stares deeply, and then breaks into a big smile after I greet him with a hearty, "Hello, Mardig!" He starts talking about a few things, but I can't make sense of what he's saying. Alzheimer's seems to have progressed quickly. Still, I listen to him with a warm smile and a lot of nods and yeses. I paraphrase some of the things he says, even though they don't make sense. This makes him feel comfortable communicating.

We walk in the hallways and talk awhile. I tell him I have a surprise for him. He smiles in anticipation. We look for a place to sit. A large empty activity room provides a quiet place to settle down. We sit side-by-side at a crescent-shaped table; Mardig is to my right.

I retrieve the cover page of the book and hand it to him. He begins reading. I'm hoping he'll make the connection between *a tribute to my father* and the author's name, his daughter—me. He doesn't say a word. Still, I know if he understood what he was reading, he would be proud, *very* proud. As he used to say, he would be happy "one of his own had made something of *him*self." (He typically referred to me as a *he*.)

He holds his hand out for the next page. I hand him the introduction. As he reads this page, a few residents come in. They walk around us. A woman sits to my left. I smile at her, and she smiles back. She's holding a small stuffed white bunny in her left hand while adoringly petting its head with her right. I think about my sister and her two bunnies.

Mardig continues to read. After a few moments, I ask, "So, what do you think?"

"Nice history," he replies, and resumes reading.

After a several more minutes pass, it appears he is reading and rereading only the bottom part of this introductory page. I ask if he has any questions.

"I'm amazed at the amount of money *he* acquired and that *he* changed from his home to the family home."

I am surprised by his response. *This is about him and yet he thinks he is reading about someone else!* He read about the $100,000 accumulated from his GE stock and about moving from his home to our home.

Just then, another resident walks in and stands inches from his right elbow. Mardig looks at the resident's side, then turns to me and says quietly in Armenian, "We should put these materials away and look at them later."

The lack of privacy in the skilled nursing facility is something I am still trying to get used to. It happens so frequently; I have little choice. How do I ask someone with Alzheimer's to go elsewhere? Each resident needs lots of nods and kindness. I've learned, even as they look over our shoulders, they don't know what they are seeing. Occasionally the staff and aides gently redirect a resident to give my father and me privacy.

I encourage Mardig to continue reading because the person by his side has moved. I then hand him the first page of the chapter, "Little Things Matter the Most."[1] Pointing to the section describing his eighty-seventh birthday, I tell him, "Mardig, this is about *your* eighty-seventh birthday party held *here*!" He starts reading.

It occurs to me this is a *rare gift*. Here I am, writing a tribute to him, and he is reading it! Why not include his remarks? I take the pages he has already read and on their blank backsides, I start writing notes before I forget. I recall how we walked the hallways and talked, what his initial reactions are to the introduction of this book, and his other comments.

He refers to what he has read in the third person. After a few minutes, I ask Mardig if he knows whose eighty-seventh birthday it was. He replies, "The two of us, I guess." He quietly reads for a bit longer and then describes it in the third person using "he" and "him."

I clarify, "Mardig, this is about you." I'm not sure he agrees.

He then reads about my mother ironing. Again, I ask whom he is reading about. "Pa," he replies, "since it's downstairs. Ma would be upstairs." *Was he recalling people based on where they were in the house?*

---

1 This, and the following quotes referring to what my father read, are from the first edition of *"Where's my shoes?"*

"Do you remember this?" I ask, wondering if he remembered my mother ironing.

"Yeah, playing with Pa's clothes, putting 'em in shape." *It was as if he were I!* "What are they doing now?" he asks.

He continues reading and sometimes makes comments. I watch him, my attention occasionally drawn to other people in the room. A woman sits in a *geri-chair*, a type of wheelchair that also reclines. She was wheeled into the room by one of the aides and positioned toward our right side. She has short, curly white hair. She's wearing a T-shirt with a message I can't read. A pale pink sheet on her lap is the object of her attention as she takes great care to fold it and then unfold it, making certain the edges line up. I watch as she repeats this action a half-dozen times. She is completely immersed in her work, never noticing me looking at her while my father reads.

My attention shifts back to Mardig. He is saying, "Unrelated situation sparking warm memories." He points to each word with his right index finger as he reads a few lines aloud. "My mother ironing . . . I remember my mother spending a lot of time each week ironing. I remember her ironing upstairs in the master bedroom of our home. I remember some warm summer days when she'd iron downstairs in the living room or the sunroom." He continues to read quietly.

After awhile he reaches the part where we are playing checkers and my mother takes his pieces. I ask, "Do you know who this is about?"

"I'm getting to it," he replies, adding, "Pa."

"Are *you* in here?" I ask, emphasizing "you."

"No."

"But you know these . . ."

". . . situations. Yeah," he completes my sentence.

He stops reading, notices the wind blowing outside, and then turns to me. "Things outside home . . . they been taken care of?"

Wow! He was aware of the windy day. "Yes."

He looks into my eyes to be sure I mean it.

He takes another page and points to a paragraph. It is in the sibling rivalry section where I wrote about our height being another source of competition. I ask, "Do you remember who this is about?"

"About Pa, because he was the earner," he answers.

He reads a short paragraph aloud: "When I think of it, it's truly amazing how differently kids grow into adults."

When he finishes, I say, "This is about your children, Mardig."

He does not reply.

In the end, he stuck with it. He read the entire manuscript I brought for him to read, seven pages in all.

If I was looking for recognition or appreciation, there was none to be given in the traditional sense. But if I wanted the rare and good fortune to see my father read my tribute to him before he died, I GOT IT!

I repeated: "Mardig, this is a book I am writing about *you*."

"It'll be interesting in years to come," he said.

CHAPTER 20

Voluntary Conservatorship

While Mardig thrives in the nursing home, my brother and sister attempt to undermine my fiduciary responsibility over our father's estate. Because I had challenged our brother's right to keep the money he questionably acquired and possibly because my sister was unhappy we did not let her have our parents' home at a steal of a price, they communicated with me through their lawyers. My brother retained high-powered attorneys in California and Wisconsin and fed both an unbalanced diet of information. He never questioned my ability to care for our father. The issue centered squarely on our father's finances.

During the two years before he moved to California, Mardig increasingly expressed concerns and feelings of helplessness to David and me. He was concerned about how my brother took his money, and he wanted to get it back. Mardig even talked with my sister and enlisted her help to draft a letter of what happened.

On the rare occasions when my sister and I spoke, we briefly touched on this topic. I, however, was in the dark as to the details, despite being asked to bear witness to an awkward confrontation several years earlier.

Only days after my mother's passing in 1993, Mardig asked me to be present when he talked with my brother regarding a "money matter." All he wanted me to do was sit and listen.

Mardig and I walked into the dining room where my brother was sitting on an old barstool, bent over an elevated glass-topped table attending to some paperwork. Greeting him by name, Mardig said, "I'd like to have a word with you."

Without looking up, my brother said, "Yeah, sure. What's up?"

I sat on a chair by the doorway leading into the kitchen while Mardig stood, waiting for his son to look at him. Mardig repeated, "Can I discuss a matter with you?"

Still without looking up, "Yeah."

"It looks like you're busy, we can talk another time."

My brother looked briefly at Mardig and, with slight irritation in his voice, said, "We can talk now. Shoot!" He then returned his attention once again to his paperwork.

Our father, the diplomat, tried to be patient and polite.

Mardig began hesitatingly. He spoke of our mother being gone now and how sad it was. My brother half listened as he continued working. Mardig described my brother: a successful business owner in his early forties, with employees, who traveled. Then Mardig described his situation: a retired man in his eighties with limited income potential. Finally, Mardig requested the money be returned.

My brother spun around on the barstool, stood up, and took two steps toward our father. Noted for his tempers, I feared the confrontation would escalate. I stood up and took one step forward.

Our father, now between us, stood his ground.

My brother did not take another step. In a raised voice, he refused to return the money, insisting it was his and that Ma had intended it for him. Incensed, he spewed forth a monologue of indignation at such a challenge to his righteousness.

I sighed and sat down. I listened to what he was saying with astonishment. Here he was, at age forty-two, still living in his father's home.

It was awkward being put in this position, especially when my father had been so private.

Each time Mardig expressed concern about money owed to him, David and I insisted he write a will reflecting his wishes. This way, there would be no question about his intentions. He'd jokingly reply, "I'm gonna live another fifteen years. What if I change my mind?"

"You can easily change it," we assured him.

He'd repeat his concern about the money and add, "I want you to remember this, because if there's any disagreement, I want you to know the truth."

It was only in preparation for the April meeting we learned the details.

While poring through Mardig's paperwork, we saw line after line, page upon page, the notes of a tortured and tormented man. He feared the house was legally his son's and his son's irritation with him would result in his eviction. He wrote of how his son would routinely ask for money when equipment and supplies were shipped to the house COD or when his son asked Mardig to accompany him shopping and then asked Mardig to pay. Mardig's still waiting to be paid back.

And then there was an issue Mardig wrote about in several places: *One day, under the pretense that [my son] wanted me to learn how to take care of Mom, he told me to be at the hospital at a given time . . . I was shepherded into a room set for conference. The individual (an attorney) asked me to sign a couple of sheets turning [a money market fund] over to [my son]. . . . In [my wife's] condition I was not in a quarreling mood as bad as she was physically . . . another contract was thrust to me. The house. Even in the charged atmosphere I could not see a reason to release the house. No explanation as to what I was to do; buy another or pay rent. When I declined, not a word from the attorney. I guess he saw the absurdity; obviously, this was not the attorney's idea. The avariciousness that [my son] displayed on this occasion was far beyond my belief. While other boys borrow, get into debt, for an education, [my son] never had that trouble.*

Except for 2-3 weeks for military exercises, [my son] has always been at home. While the girls received a pittance by comparison, [my son] took the whole pie and even picked up the crumbs.

My father was so distraught he was grasping at straws. We even found a letter he drafted to a Milwaukee alderwoman.

Meanwhile, his brother who I visited in Illinois, said Mardig discussed this situation with him and had retained an attorney in an effort to get his money back. "Brenda, your brother needs to return that money. It's not his. It's your father's."

As my father loses his abilities to Alzheimer's disease, there are moments he is lucid. It is during these moments when I can't stop wondering, What if he's aware? What if Mardig knows what's really going on?

Others have asked the same thing. One caregiver asks during a support group meeting, "What if I sell my mother's home and later she becomes aware and insists on moving back?" We nervously chuckle, because each of us has wondered this. Common sense says otherwise, but it's still a concern.

David and I worked hard to get the home Mardig bought in 1952 ready to sell. My sister, brother, and I selected a few items of sentimental value and then I arranged to sell or donate the rest, depositing the proceeds in his estate.

What if one day we're sitting together and talking, and Mardig sits up and exclaims in very clear terms, "I'm finished here. I want to go home now."

Uh-uhhh . . . hmm, I don't know exactly how to tell you this, but nine months after we moved you to California, we sold your home in Milwaukee.

"You, *what*?" we imagine him asking. Except, he would be more diplomatic. "Why would *you* sell *my* house?"

And then we would be speechless, feeling utter embarrassment at what we had done.

Months earlier, Mardig was aware. When he first moved to California, he was aware he was forgetting. "I don't remember the English language like I used to," he'd say. I'd encourage him to speak in Armenian. He would chuckle and add, "I'm forgetting. The words don't come as easily."

But now, what if he is truly aware? What if this was all an act? What if he's been studying how we will react?

Yes, I realize this seems farfetched, but I can't stop wondering.

By June 1997, with no more communication between my siblings and me, my concerns intensify. Fearing issues would remain after our father's passing, and that the power of attorney did not give me the scope of powers I needed given the contentious circumstances, I looked for certainty. There were at least a dozen issues that had to be resolved before our father died, including a major one for David and me—*stress*. We distilled these into a handful:

1. Ignore the sizable sum of money my brother obtained from Mardig and potentially be held liable by my sister after our father's passing. She could argue I did not exercise adequate fiduciary responsibility over his estate. *We really had no idea what she would do. She didn't reply to most of our inquiries, including those from the attorney.*

2. Proceed with my father's wishes to have my brother return the funds to the estate, including a five-figure promissory note drafted in 1993 and due in 1994 that was still not paid back.

3. If, given Mardig's age and health, his estate and monthly income are ample enough to pay for his care, emergencies, and future tax liabilities; provide cash gifts to my sister and me now in order to reduce the estate tax and the disparity among beneficiaries. *But what if my father lives a long time and needs these funds for his care? I could not imagine my sister willingly returning the money, much less getting anything back from my brother.*

4. Receive compensation since I was shouldering much of the responsibility and had essentially given up my career while handling all these unexpected complexities and details. In 1997

alone, approximately 1,000 hours were devoted to Mardig's affairs—a half-time job, and he was in a skilled nursing facility!

5. Find options to deal with the stress David and I were experiencing related to Mardig's paperwork and estate-related matters.

We went to the attorney with these issues and asked if a conservatorship would give us more certainty. He advised we continue documenting the details and extend an olive branch to my brother and sister with a simpler and less costly approach: a *Consent and Settlement Agreement* and *Mutual Release* document, drafted with the help of David Cohn, Mardig's Milwaukee attorney. Attorney Cohn drafted the initial power of attorney based on our assumption that my father's affairs were simple and straightforward. It offered no direction for the issues we now faced. Attorney Cohn's humor went a long way to help reduce tensions. "Yes, we'll take this one step at a time. First the olive branch, next the glove, and finally the bare fist." His fighting spirit gave us strength when we felt powerless. My stress level skyrocketed as we drafted, revised, and edited the key issues of this document with both attorneys. I wanted to make sure this document was drafted in such a way that at least my sister would sign it. I needed predictability.

Mardig could have avoided all this if he created a legal document in advance outlining his wishes.

While my brother insisted he was entitled to our father's money, my sister remained uncharacteristically quiet. I was surprised, considering she complained about Mardig's early morning visits and of not getting anything after our mother died. David and I reasoned she would jump at this opportunity because we included gifting provisions to equalize the estate among the three beneficiaries. I hoped my brother would sign it, because the extended olive branch was reasonable—he would not have to immediately return a major portion of the funds. Instead, it would be deducted from his inheritance if any money remained. I also assumed they would sign the document because, thanks to the rising stock market during the time I managed Mardig's accounts, his estate had grown significantly.

Neither signed the document.

My stress level remained high. I needed assurance what we were doing would not come to haunt us later. I kept detailed records, questioned the accountant and the attorneys about every move I made. The only thing I did contrary to their advice, given Mardig's advanced age, was to leave most of his assets in equities. Being more risk-tolerant, I took this calculated risk and was ultimately rewarded with higher returns.

Meanwhile, David and I scoured my father's papers and David grew more bitter. "I hate your brother for what he did to your father; for how he treated Mardig. He's going to pay for it. We will take him to court. We will make him pay back everything, plus interest!"

I felt uncomfortable when David talked like this. "David. David." I said, trying to interrupt his tirade. "Let's see what the attorneys can do."

I didn't mind a good fight, especially with help from an attorney like David Cohn. But Mardig didn't write a will despite our earlier requests of him to do so. We could have avoided most of these headaches. Reality's sting was painful. *Why should I pick up the pieces when he didn't even plan for them? Why do I have to do all the dirty work? Let it be! My sister is not even responding to our correspondence. What should I care? My brother won't sue, he's the one who benefited!*

"Brenda, remember why you went to the attorney in the first place. You want predictability. Even though your sister is not talking to you, she can come after you later," David reminded me.

"Yeah, yeah," I said. "Okay, we'll try to get a conservatorship. It seems to be the only way. Gee, when the first attorney told us to get one, I concluded he was trying to make us spend money needlessly. Now look at us. I should have taken his advice."

"Remember, Mardig wanted his money back. Let the courts force your brother to pay back what he took."

"Yeah, but the attorney doesn't think a conservatorship is

necessary. Remember? He said we could simply get an addendum to our POA or a temporary conservatorship. I don't actually remember what he said exactly."

"He did say, 'There are no guarantees,'" reminded David.

"Yeah, that annoys me. Why do we even need attorneys if there are no guarantees? They're supposed to protect us. Why did we even get into this mess in the first place?" I continued.

"Because your father would've died if we had left him in Milwaukee. He's alive, and he's enjoying himself . . . even though he doesn't know where he is."

"No, I don't mean that! Why did we take on this financial mess? Look at all the time we spent on that *Consent* document. For what? They didn't even sign it!"

"Brenda, you want predictability. This is what it takes," David responded.

"I really don't want to get the courts involved."

"I don't either, and I'm sure your father doesn't want take this to court. But remember, he did want his money back. And your brother was mean to him. That was nasty what he pulled on your father in the hospital. You need the court's decision. Then your brother and sister can't say anything."

We amicably terminated our relationship with the California attorney. After more than a year of helping us lay the groundwork and responding to my sister's and brother's attorneys, by early 1998 we needed someone to help us take the next step. Growing increasingly concerned about avoiding litigation after my father's passing, David and I needed someone who would be willing to stand in court and to fight if necessary; "to put the gloves on," as Attorney Cohn said.

I received referrals for eight attorneys. I rated each according to criteria important to me at this stage—successful litigation experience, forthright, detail oriented, prompt follow-up, and certified. I interviewed three at great length via telephone to get a feeling for how we'd interact. Then I received a last-minute referral for another attorney, who I also interviewed. I chose her. With an office fifty-five miles away, this petite middle-aged attorney was in hyper-drive. Constantly on the go, she'd juggle two and three clients at one time. While in her office, she'd take a call from a client. While talking with that client, another client would call. She'd handle these calls and then return her attention to us. Although impressive, it was frustrating to keep her focused. Then again, when I phoned, she'd answer my call while another client waited in her office. She was the attorney we needed to take us to the next level.

In the summer of 1998, we finally petitioned the court for conservatorship. We attended a hearing in the fall. Since my sister and brother had been unresponsive and uncooperative, we would get the court's ruling on the scope of my fiduciary and healthcare responsibilities. Unbelievably, I had to first be bonded for the value of my father's estate. It is the law. I considered this money wasted.

A month later, I was granted conservatorship over the "person and estate of Martin Avadian." My brother and sister didn't object.

As we did in 1996 and 1997, after we learned of my father's different accounts, we sent letters to a dozen places notifying them of the change of status—now from power of attorney to conservator. *Just what we need, more paperwork.* We had to re-title all the accounts showing "Brenda Avadian, Conservator of the Person and Estate of Martin Avadian." I had to sign all his documents this way. We also notified the skilled nursing facility, the local hospital where my father would be taken in case of an emergency, and my father's doctor.

I made sure to do one important thing after learning from fellow caregiver Patti's experience with her husband. When she was appointed Ralph's conservator, she never received the authority to give consent for medical treatment. Consequently, her beloved Ralph languished in a near comatose state while Patti fought with his children from a previous marriage to allow him to go in peace. I heeded her advice and petitioned the Superior Court in California for special orders regarding dementia, including the exclusive authority to give consent for medical treatment. This meant before my father was treated or prescribed psychotropic medications, the doctor had to discuss it with me. I could also withhold consent for medical treatment when it did not seem necessary. Since I did not have medical knowledge to make informed decisions, I questioned each proposed treatment until I understood why the doctor advised it and its perceived benefits. This did have one added benefit. After all my questioning, the doctors really thought before they suggested something. In this way, I served as my father's caring advocate. *We all need one!*

After being appointed conservator, the accountant helped us put together an *Inventory and Appraisement* of Mardig's assets. The accountant we retained had been doing a great job of producing annual accountings that we voluntarily sent to my sister and brother. Within the year, we petitioned the court to approve the accounting, which it did.

Step by step we worked through the issues I raised more than a year earlier. Each time we petitioned the court, copies of our petition were mailed to all of Mardig's heirs and attorneys, including a copy sent to Mardig at the skilled nursing facility. I did not like this, because of the sensitivity of the issues we were petitioning. But, as with everything else, we learned to cope.

When we finally went to court for a ruling on my brother's right to the money, a battle erupted. Up until then, we were progressing relatively smoothly. From Wisconsin, my brother retained a major Los Angeles law firm to represent him in court. My attorney started getting cold feet. "I can't stand up to a large law firm that has an entire staff to work on a case, Brenda. It's just me and my paralegal!"

I gulped. After everything we'd been through, I didn't want to look for another attorney. Not now. I was confident we would win—with her legal knowledge and experience and the information I had. "You can, trust me. I know we will win."

"I don't know," she said.

I had not seen her doubt herself before. She had been confident we'd get the court's approval each step of the way. But this was different. "I have damaging information regarding my brother."

"Let's see it."

"No, I can't . . . not yet."

"Brenda, if you want me to win and you want me to represent you, you have to give me all the information you have."

"I can't," I hesitated. "It's just too embarrassing."

"Do you think your brother cares? Look at the false information he's feeding his attorneys."

"Yeaaah, I know. But . . . hmmm. SIGH. Okay. I'll give you pieces of it at a time."

"Why pieces?"

"Because I know my father would not want me to share our family's ugliness."

"I understand, but let me decide. I need to see it, now!"

I relented. "All right. I will get it together and send it to you as soon as possible."

"Good. And Brenda, I'll review the documents and show them to your brother's attorneys. Maybe we won't even have to present them in court."

"That would be good," I sighed.

During this time, spanning over a year, no one had represented my sister in court. Just my husband, our attorney, my brother's attorney, and I went to court each time.

Then a message arrived. *Both* my sister and brother wanted our father's assets to be managed by a professional trustee. *What? After all I had done, this is what I get? How could they?* I hated them for erecting this obstacle. I fumed all the way home from the courthouse. The following day, after a good night's rest, I had calmed down. *This might not be so bad. Someone else can handle the day-to-day details.* But, I couldn't let go entirely.

By the middle of 2000, I resigned my responsibility as conservator so the trustee could take over. However, I insisted on serving in an advisory capacity. The trustee agreed to this with the written agreement the trust company will not be held accountable for losses. My brother and sister did not object to this arrangement.

More paperwork! We sent letters and filled out forms for each of the institutions in order to transfer Mardig's assets into the trust. *When will this end?*

The savings bonds would be a problem. Even though my father regularly purchased bonds over the years, providing steady accumulation of wealth with little risk of loss, they involved a lot of record keeping. David kept track of which ones stopped or were about to stop earning interest. I had to find time to go to the safety deposit box, remove those bonds, and sign each one with that lengthy conservatorship signature. If there were too many, the bank would have to send them to the U.S. Department of Treasury to process. Either way, the funds were then deposited into the trust account. But this was not all.

Mardig still held GE stock certificates he bought years ago. My mother's name appeared on some of them. In order to transfer these into Mardig's trust account, we had to change the record of ownership. We ordered a certified copy of my mother's death certificate from Milwaukee and then sent it and the stock certificates to GE to have them re-title Mardig as the owner.

Eventually, both the correctly named stock certificates and bonds were transferred to the trustee. David sent an itemized list of the bonds' face value, date, type, and serial number. The trustee laid out a plan to cash them in to minimize the tax burden in any given year.

The trustee wanted to reallocate Mardig's assets and put some in mutual funds managed by their parent organization. I wanted them to retain my father's stock holdings because they were still growing.

Meanwhile, my sister and brother never commented about how I cared for our father. Their comments focused on how I was managing his estate.

We still needed the court's decision on my brother's right to keep the questionably acquired funds. I dragged my feet on presenting additional proof to my attorney. Our father's journals were incriminating and I struggled with airing our family's bad side. *Is this why Mardig stopped short of taking his son to court?* At the same time, I couldn't believe how strongly my brother's attorneys were pressuring my attorney to give up my fight.

I finally put a package together, and, at her request, included transcripts of our April family meeting. Typing those transcripts was an ordeal I hope to never relive. Too embarrassed to show this kind of information to a professional transcriber, who could have done it infinitely faster, I suffered and cursed through each hour and day I typed, rewound the cassette tape and played it again, typed some more. I repeated this more than a hundred times.

During the court hearing, my brother's attorneys rejected the argument that the funds belonged to my father. Immediately my attorney requested a trial. My brother's attorney then asked for a private meeting with my attorney. A few minutes later, they emerged from the judge's chambers. My attorney had presented the documents to my brother's attorney. He agreed the funds were my father's. The court ruled likewise.

Relieved this was behind me, I walked out of the courtroom with my head held high. Mardig won. I could imagine only a few things worse than that experience.

Just to be sure, I asked my attorney, "Does this mean I don't have to worry about my sister or brother raising issues after my father dies?"

"Unfortunately, Brenda, there are no guarantees," she said.

I wish she didn't say that!

CHAPTER 21

Treasuring Small Moments

It's ten minutes to six, twenty minutes into dinnertime, when David and I visit Mardig at the skilled nursing facility. We walk into the lobby and the receptionist greets us with a warm hello. We ask her to let us into the secured area of the facility where the residents live. We hear the now-familiar *buzz* that electronically releases the lock, and we turn the levered doorknob and walk inside. We stand for a moment by the door, surveying the place. Three halls extend in different directions; one directly ahead, another to the left, and the third, to our right. We start walking ahead when one of the Armenian aides who spends time with my father informs us Mardig is finishing his dinner in the dining room. She encourages us to join him.

Looking forward to a new experience, we walk toward the dining room. Residents' families are discouraged from visiting during mealtimes because, as it was once explained to us, the residents get distracted by new faces and get up without finishing their meals.

We hesitate at the doorway to the dining room, looking for Mardig. One of the activity coordinators whose smile and attention Mardig greatly enjoys, approaches us and asks, "Are you looking for Martin?"

"Yes."

She graciously motions us to come in. "Come with me. He's back here, eating his dinner."

We follow her to a row of tables in the back where we learn Mardig likes to sit; especially since he's usually one of the last to show up for his meals. Residents who arrive earlier take the seats near the entrance.

"Marteen!" she exclaims, accentuating the long "e" sound. "Your daughter is here to see you!"

We thank her and she smiles and walks away to take care of another resident. Mardig looks up at me and then David. His eyes open wide.

"Oh, am I glad to see you!" he says, clasping his hands together. "Am I glad you came!" With this enthusiastic greeting, we sit down. I sit next to Mardig and David sits next to me.

"What did you come here for?" he asks.

"To see you!" we reply, with big smiles.

"Me?" he says, amazed he is the reason for our visit.

"Yes, you!" I exclaim, kiddingly nudging his shoulder.

"Great!" he says and returns to his meal.

He eats his food and minds his own business. This is good. At least he is eating. David and I talk a little about our day. Another resident sitting across from Mardig grabs our attention.

"Do you know where they parked my car?"

"Hmmm," I wonder how to respond because it's hard to know what he's thinking.

"Did they park it by LaSalle and Michigan?"

"LaSalle and Michigan in Chicago?" I ask, hoping he will feel understood.

His eyes light up for an instant and he nods.

"Yes," I say, "they parked it right where you asked them to."

"Good," he says. "Well, I'm going to go get it then."

I look at David and ask, "What is this? Is everyone from Chicago?"

My father lived in Chicago before moving to Milwaukee. Since moving into the nursing facility he often spoke of places he remembered in Chicago. One of his roommates in the facility was also from Chicago. He told stories of how Mardig (his imaginary brother) and he used to play ball when they were kids. They called Mardig, *The Kid*, he'd say. Even though this was not true, I wanted to believe they knew each other. It was nice to know he believed they had something in common. As confused as people's minds get with this disease, any bit of familiarity, whether real or imagined, comforts them.

We observed Mardig slowly eat his dinner. He reached for the white bread on his tray. His left hand shook a little as he picked up the sandwich. He carefully wedged his right index finger in between the slices to see what was inside. He pulled out an oily finger and then took a big bite out of the soft buttered bread.

I couldn't get beyond the way my father looked as he sat there, hunched over the table, his extended hand slightly shaking as he grasped a spoonful of food and carefully balanced it as he brought it toward his mouth. We sat watching him, occasionally chatting, but mostly watching him.

"Doesn't he look cute?" I asked David.

"Uhhh, I suppose so."

Where did that come from? I rarely referred to Mardig as cute. Yet, there was something cute about him just now. He looked a bit helpless. After all, what would he do if this nice meal were not prepared for him? He couldn't fend for himself anymore. I sat there, thankful he received such well-balanced meals and that he was still able to eat them on his own. It's only a matter of time before he will have to be helped, because he will have forgotten how to feed himself.

As he ate, his mouth almost touched the dishes on his tray. He had to raise his elbow shoulder height to clear the tray when reaching for his food. With trembling hands, he gently reached out and spooned or forked whatever he wanted. He liked soft food best; mashed potatoes, white bread, or stuffing. Soft sweet foods were even better!

David and I quietly watched him eat. Occasionally we looked at the other residents and at the aides who were removing trays of food left by the residents.

When he was finished, Mardig reached over for a napkin and

carefully wiped his mouth. He neatly folded his napkin and placed it on his tray. I handed him a toothpick; he liked one after a meal. Toothpicks were *contraband* in the facility, since a misplaced toothpick could poke a resident. He glanced at me when I handed him the toothpick. He took it, used it briefly, and then placed it toward the back of his tray. He stood, picked up his tray, and handed it to the aide who smiled and thanked him. She looked over to us and said, "Martin always does this. He hands us his tray."

He then turned to us and said as politely as he could muster, "Well, it was my pleasure to join you for dinner. Thank you." Then he turned around and quickly walked toward the doors exiting the dining room.

I sat there with my mouth hanging open. I was surprised at what had happened. My father had no clue who we were. And then David and I began to laugh. *What else could we do in a situation like this? It was truly comical. My father had no idea.*

The more of Mardig this disease takes away, the closer we look at seemingly insignificant moments in order to hold onto what remains of him. These are what we'll remember when he's no longer with us.

When Mardig was admitted to the facility, he'd worry about money. "I don't want to eat. Who's going to pay for it?"

"It's already paid for."

"Who paid for it?" he'd ask, genuinely curious who was paying his way.

"We did," we'd sometimes say.

"I'll pay you back."

"That's alright," we'd say, trying to comfort him. He was really paying for the meals and his stay at the facility. He didn't believe he had enough money and we didn't want him to worry. David and I decided to try another response the next time he asked.

"The government is paying for this."

"It is? Why is the government paying for me?"

"Because you're retired and this is the benefit they provide." *What does one say? Sure, it's a lie. But with his memory impaired, it was important to make him feel comfortable.*

"Good," he said happily.

He'd sometimes ask us for a dollar. Other times, he'd ask, "Do you have any money on you?"

"Yes."

"Can I have some?"

"How much?"

"How much have you got?"

I'd open my wallet and show him the twenties and tens inside. He'd grab a ten and say, "Thanks. This'll last me for a while. I'll pay you back." Then he'd stuff the money into his pants pocket. As the months passed, he'd ask for less money, mostly change for a phone call.

As Mardig lost hold of reality, he created his own world. He asked about Ma and Pa. Sometimes Ma was his mother; other times she was his wife (my mother). We were unclear because he'd just ask, "Are you going to see Ma?" "How's Ma doing?" "How's Pa doing?"

Months earlier, we'd tell him the truth. We couldn't lie. "Your parents died a long time ago," I'd remind him. He'd look depressed and stop talking. His wife was alive and so were his parents, at least in his world. We didn't know what to do. David tried using logic.

"How old are you, Mardig?"

"Ohhh, I guess . . . seventy . . . eighty?" he'd inquire, looking at David for confirmation.

"Your parents would have to be near one hundred if they were still alive!"

My father would look amazed and we'd all laugh, knowing this was impossible since our family typically lived only into their seventies and eighties.

There would be silence and then Mardig would change the subject.

Each time we'd visit, he'd ask the same questions.

One day, I asked the support group about honesty and our loved ones. This must have been one of those difficult questions, because they hesitated to respond. The few caregivers who did have an opinion were divided between lying and telling the truth. I confidently shared my opinion: honesty was important in the caregiving relationship. I went on and on about integrity and how we had the responsibility to our loved ones to tell them the truth. Upon hearing my confident assertions, no one else spoke about the issue. After the meeting, Jeanne, a nurse and caregiver to her mother, pulled me aside and asked me to consider something. "Brenda, given your father's forgetfulness, each time you tell him his parents and wife are gone, you are making him relive the loss again. Realize he doesn't remember they died. It's a surprise to him each time."

I sighed, not liking what I was hearing.

"Brenda, I know you like to tell the truth. If you have a hard time lying then just deflect the comment and bring up pleasant memories of your mom when he talks about her."

"Aww, alright, I'll try," I said unconvincingly. "Jeanne?"

"Yeah?"

"Thanks."

The next time Mardig talked about Ma, my mother, I asked him if he remembered how we used to pack picnics for brunch at the lakefront on Sundays. He smiled and said he didn't remember but was amazed I did. "You really enjoyed those, didn't you?" I nodded my head. It worked!

At the next meeting, I thanked Jeanne and began recommending others use the same deflection technique. It's hard because we want to be honest. Yet, by being truthful we sometimes hurt an impaired person. I've heard some refer to this as *therapeutic lying*.

Each time I was with my father, I deflected his comments about people who were no longer with us. It took some practice because I couldn't resist my old habit of telling the truth. But it was working and he was feeling so much better about the people he talked about.

I continued going through the things from Mardig's house in Milwaukee, all his notes and his journals. In some he wrote: "I'm writing this so I don't forget." Even while he lived with us, he'd take notes to make sense of his world. Sometimes, I saw it as a desperate measure to hang onto reality.

His methodical qualities made me smile. As I was cleaning the closet of his room in our home, I ran across some Halloween decorations. One was a three-foot coiled rubber snake. He tightly wrapped the snake with packing thread so it wouldn't uncoil. He even took pains to tie a half bow so you could pull one end of the thread to easily untie his handiwork.

While cleaning out his desk in Milwaukee, I found an audiocassette tape painstakingly hand-wrapped around an empty orange-colored spool of correcto-ribbon used on electric typewriters. *What was his plan for this? Why would he take time to carefully hand wrap magnetic tape in this fashion?*

Everything had to be wrapped, boxed, and put away. And he'd say, "I'll look at it later."

In our daily lives, moments sneak by, barely noticed. It's hard to know what to keep as I go through my father's things. *What will have meaning for me tomorrow? I may experience something different in life that will lead to another insight into my father.* I try not to throw away too much, even though I don't like collecting things. I don't want to be a slave to my possessions; especially after I saw how much my parents' things weighed them down.

Sorting through Mardig's paperwork did yield a few treasures. When Mardig was in his thirties he signed his name *M. Avadian.* Coincidentally, I made the decision to sign my name the same way in my late twenties; the initial of my first name and my full last name. The amount of paperwork I had to sign, including multi-part carbonless pages, made this a necessity. Stabbing pain frequently invaded my right wrist; so, I reasoned, if I had less to write, it would not hurt as much. I was surprised to see Mardig had signed his name this way. In his forties, he went back to signing his complete name. *I continue to sign my name using my first initial.*

Up until his sixties, Mardig was a meticulous record keeper. I was pleased to find the hospital bill for my birth. It cost $150 to bring me into this world in 1959. He also recorded when I had chicken pox. Perhaps the accompanying 106° fever damaged my nerves, resulting in my deaf left ear.

Mardig kept records of his finances. He followed a conservative and low-risk approach to his investments. Opting for U.S. savings bonds, certificate of deposits, and treasury funds, he rebuffed my suggestion in the mid-1980s to invest in the stock and options markets. He did buy stock in a railroad company and a couple others in his earlier years though. However, I did not find any record of the results of these early investments.

Among his papers I found a document entitled, Fitch Stock Summary, April 1943 issue, by Harris, Upham, & Company. This document published stock prices during the years of the Great Depression. Surprisingly, AT&T's prices ranged from a high of $310.25 to a low of $70.25 from 1929 to 1942. General Electric's range was equally surprising from $100.75 to $8.50! IBM, $255 to $52.50! Accounting for all the stock splits during the following sixty years, I can't imagine what these stocks would be worth today. Commodities were also listed. No precious metals were traded at that time. But black pepper was a listed commodity in 1942. What a treasure!

When I think about my father these are the small moments I treasure. After all, the little things are what make lasting memories.

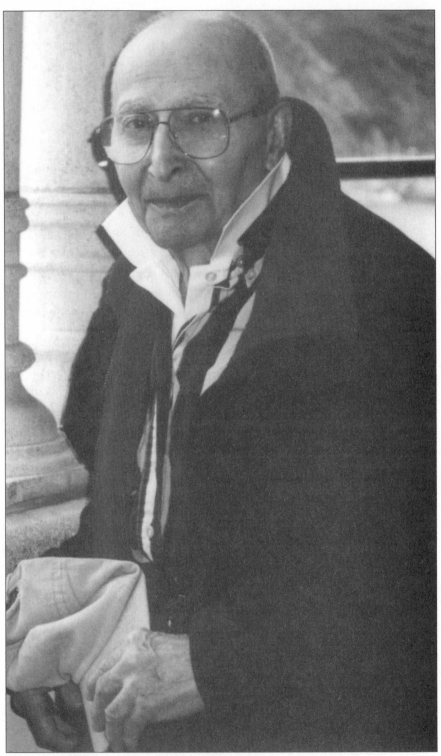

Martin Avadian at Catalina Island, March 1997.

FIVE

A Seed is Planted

CHAPTER 22

Will Mardig See the New Millennium?

Mardig thrives in the skilled nursing facility. In August, we bring him home to celebrate his eighty-eighth birthday and my thirty-ninth. David has baked a double-layer carrot cake topped with cream cheese icing. I've added colorful decorations including "Happy 88th Birthday, Mardig." Our caregiving family and friends have joined us to eat, talk, and laugh as we watch Mardig open gifts and read his birthday cards. Betty, a caregiver for her late husband, moves next to Mardig to help him read his cards. As he reads the stack of fifteen cards over and over again, Betty asks, "Martin, what are you doing?"

He looks at her, smiles, and exclaims, "Wow! I've got a lot of cards and I don't even know these people!" We laugh.

It's time to serve the cake. We place two number 8 candles on top of the cake and light them. We show Mardig his cake and ask him to make a wish then blow out his candles. After he blows out the candles, I hand him a piece of cake. He quietly says, "I wish my balls were shaped that way." I can't believe what I hear and ask others what he said. Sure enough, he expressed his wish! We laugh heartily. Mardig smiles. The comment is so uncharacteristic of my father. Yet as Alzheimer's wreaks havoc on his brain, the roundness of the two eights on the cake must remind him of his male anatomy.

Mardig's birthday celebration is bittersweet. We are happy he is alive yet we are sad he does not understand what we're celebrating. But, he is having fun and this is important.

He is not on any medications and his weight remains steady between 118 and 120 pounds. He has slowed down noticeably and is more confused, but he still flirts with the female aides and any woman who smiles and is kind to him.

Mardig no longer recognizes David's and my relationship to him. When we visit, he walks past us. Our friends think this must be hard for us to accept. I can't explain it, but it's not. We accept Mardig as he is. Sure, we prefer he recognize us and call us by name, as he did one afternoon during a moment of lucidity. As we watched him walk away, he turned abruptly, looked at me, and asked, "Hey, Brenda, who was that person who was going to take care of . . .?" I was astonished. For three months he had no idea who I was, and in this one brief moment, he called me by name. He knew I was his daughter!

Most of the time, David and I can't make sense of our conversations with him. We ask about his day, his children, his wife, and his work at General Electric. He responds about something else, like fixing the car, or waiting for imaginary people. He even asks if we saw Ma and Pa (his parents).

There are times Mardig's incontinence is problematic. It began when he was living with us. Soon after he was in the nursing home, he started to wear protective underwear. He does not feel the need to use the bathroom until it is too late to avoid an accident. Sometimes David and I help Mardig use the bathroom and, with a staff member's assistance, will clean and change him.

No matter how respectfully we assist Mardig, he still needs help going to the bathroom. I would not wish this indignity upon anyone. Yet, I also realize we are fortunate there institutions and caregivers to help our loved ones live their remaining years with as much dignity as possible.

As Alzheimer's continues to ravage Mardig's brain, he loses his balance more often. According to the staff, he loves to walk until he's exhausted. They encourage him to sit in a geri-chair for required periods of rest.

Months pass. David and I continue visiting him once or twice a week. Mardig does relatively well. I wonder if he will survive until the year 2000, the goal he set at the kitchen table of his Milwaukee home.

Then the calls begin.

"Mr. Avadian fell earlier today. We've ordered an x-ray."

"Mr. Avadian fell last night, but he seems to be doing well. He doesn't seem to be in any pain. The doctor will see him in the morning."

The calls about Mardig falling are more frequent, and I grow increasingly concerned. I don't want him to break a hip. At his age, recovery would take forever. "I'm really concerned about him breaking something. What proactive measures are you taking to prevent his falls?"

"We are scheduling him for periods of rest."

"You've tried this with the geri-chair and it doesn't seem to be working. How about putting him in a wheelchair?" *I hate this idea, but I don't want Mardig to break a bone.*

"We can't."

"Why?"

"Because he is ambulatory. The state will not allow us to place residents in a wheelchair who are still able to walk."

Disappointed after hearing *policy* instead of a custom *solution* for my father, I ask, "Well, what policies does the State of California have if my father falls and breaks his hip?"

We debate policy versus my concern. *I understand the state wants residents to walk as long as possible. But given my father's falls, I am more concerned for his quality of life after he breaks something.* They finally agree to put Mardig in a wheelchair and schedule periods of supervised walks.

In December 1999, I receive a letter saying the skilled nursing facility has changed ownership. *Hurray!* New management takes over. *Yes!* It is now called the Antelope Valley Care Center (AVCC). *What a relief! What a difference!* Unlike the former administrator, the new one spends time among the residents and always smiles. He even attends our bi-weekly caregiver meetings, shares information, and notes family members' feedback on how to improve resident care.

We meet the new owner one afternoon when he drives up with staff members from his Los Angeles office to perform for the residents. With singers, a keyboardist, and a tambourine, the AVCC residents are entertained with songs they remember from many years ago. The group sings and plays gospel music and some popular tunes.

What a wonderful time. Residents who appear unaware are filled with the spirit of the music. Those who don't usually speak, sing along. Others, who shuffle aimlessly along the halls, get up to dance. Their fancy dance steps mesmerize me. Mardig sits in his chair with tears in his eyes. I ask, "Mardig, what's wrong?"

"The music . . . nice," he says, and smiles.

Despite the tears, it is a joyous occasion!

I used to find Mardig sitting in a chair by the station desk, where the staff gathers to update residents' charts. They'd keep an eye on him. This was good. These days he sits in a wheelchair. I can't bear to see him like this. *It's the beginning of the end.* I don't like looking down at him, so I sit in a chair so that we are eye level. Sometimes David and I race with Mardig. I hold onto Mardig while David and I run down an empty hallway. When we get to the end, he is smiling like a child pulled in a wagon. We also walk with Mardig, holding his arms to prevent him from falling.

As he wished, Mardig made it! He lived to see the year 2000—the unofficial millennium celebrated around the world. We remind him, "Mardig, this was your goal, to make it to the year 2000!" He smiles. He doesn't understand the significance anymore.

I am happy he is here with us. People ask how much longer I think Mardig will live. I don't know. A few years ago I wasn't sure he'd survive until March 1998. He made it, though; he's alive. Besides, Mardig is not ready to give up on life, and honestly, I'm not prepared to see him go. When that time comes, it will be my next challenge.

Calls continue about Mardig falling. He falls out of his wheelchair, out of bed, and when being transferred from the wheelchair to the toilet or to his bed. Something's wrong. I bring up the topic of his falling with the staff during my visits and with management during the care plan meeting. We arrive at a workable solution. So, I am annoyed when I receive another call.

"Mr. Avadian fell."

"Again? How? Isn't he in his wheelchair?"

"He tried to get out of the wheelchair. We think he reached forward and then fell over."

How disappointing! Even I've seen him reach down attempting to touch the floor or the cuffs on his pants. "Doesn't the staff watch him?"

"Well, this time he fell in his room."

"We need to do something for him. What do you suggest?"

"Use a posey on him."

"A what?"

"A posey, a restraint to prevent him from falling out of his wheelchair."

I let out a long sigh. "Okay. Let's do it. I don't want him to break anything."

Mardig's taking bigger steps toward the end.

As the disease grips more of Mardig's brain, he withdraws. He sits in a stupor, with little expression. We miss seeing his smiling face and hearing his laughter.

By late 2000, I ask about *happy meds*. Mardig's doctor is not amused by my choice of words for antidepressants, but I want quality of life for my ninety-year-old father. Anyone who lives this long deserves to be happy and comfortable. *He needs happy meds.*

A psychiatrist visits Mardig and then prescribes an antidepressant.

While Mardig descends into late-stage Alzheimer's, our white cat, Djermag, diverts our attention. She has advanced stomach cancer. We explore options, even surgery. It is too late. Days pass and she stops getting up when we open a can of cat food. For two days and nights, we help keep her warm with a heater, heating pad, and blankets. Then, on the third day, one predawn December morning, she expels fresh blood. The veterinarian warned us this would signal the end.

We take her to the animal emergency hospital. The vet places anesthetic on her forepaw, sedates her, and then inserts an IV for the euthanasia, while David holds her backside and I hold her head. She looks at me, as if to say, "It's okay, I am at peace." I believe her. Her eyes close and her warm body relaxes as she begins her long rest.

We hold her. As her body cools, we shape her into her favorite sleeping position, and place her in her bed. We bring Djermag home so her two adopted sisters can spend time with her before we bury her.

Is this preparation for my father's passing?

I grow more convinced the psychiatrist and medication are not helping Mardig. There's no sign of improvement during the first six weeks. I wonder if Mardig's getting all his medication. I jokingly tease the staff, "Have you been taking some of my father's *happy pills*?"

They laugh, "Some days, we sure could use them!"

The psychiatrist's monthly visits are not frequent enough to observe the small changes we see. His notes on Mardig's medical records don't agree with what the staff and I observe. Mardig is either the same or getting worse.

I get another call. Mardig has fallen out of bed and injured himself. Despite the raised rails on both sides of his bed, he climbs over them or crawls out from the foot of his bed. The nurse orders a weight-sensing electronic bed monitor to be placed under his sheets. An alarm will sound each time Mardig moves off the sensor. Given Mardig's slower pace, staff will have enough time to get to his room before he falls. This works for a while—until Mardig falls out of bed again. The staff is not promptly responding to the alarms. Sometimes they forget to turn on the bed monitor after helping him into bed.

During one of the caregiver support meetings at the facility, I ask the administrator what can be done to make sure staff responds to each alarm and remembers to turn on the bed monitor. He says the monitor is a new system for the facility and agrees to train all the staff members who work with my father.

At a quarterly care plan meeting I gently reiterate to management the need for staff to respond to each alarm and make sure the monitor is turned on when my father is in bed; otherwise the technology is useless.

I ask about a couple of new behaviors, teeth grinding and holding onto things. Mardig's been clenching his jaw and grinding his teeth with such a force I fear he will crush his own teeth. They schedule him to be visited by the dentist the next time he comes up to see patients. I request the dentist check and clean Mardig's teeth every quarter instead of semi-annually since he has stopped brushing his teeth. I ask why Mardig grabs and holds onto something, with fingers frozen stiff and impossible to pry open. The nurse wonders if it might be due to the antidepressant and the disease's progress. I ask how long the aides help Mardig walk each day. I appreciate they are still making him walk, because it's good for his circulation. Finally, after seeing no improvement, I ask to have the medications and the psychiatric visits stopped. They agree. By the ninth week, Mardig is no longer taking an antidepressant.

∞

Amazingly, Mardig survives to see the new millennium (2001). But his walk through Alzheimer's seems to be nearing the end. Each time there is a change in Mardig's condition, I get a call. Starting January 2001, the calls come more frequently.

"Brenda, your father is anemic. His red-blood cell level is low. There's occult blood in his stool."

Each time they phone, I panic. *This is it, he's dying!*

We talk for twenty minutes, I ask many questions.

"Mr. Avadian's doctor suggests if you want more information to follow-up with a gastroenterologist who will look at the stool samples and possibly recommend a colonoscopy."

I immediately send a detailed e-mail to other caregivers asking how they've handled a similar situation. *We caregivers know, by pooling our knowledge, we sometimes have more information than busy doctors!*

Nearly every caregiver writes about the physical strain on Mardig to prepare for a colonoscopy: the need to fast, having an enema to clean out the colon, and the anesthesia during the procedure. One caregiver summarizes it best, "If he's not in pain, let nature take its course."

After a week of making phone calls and sending and receiving e-mails, I give the AVCC my decision. With his doctor's recommendation, Mardig is to be given iron supplements and I will bring in soymilk (I recall reading something about it helping those with anemia).

Another call comes from the AVCC.

"Brenda? We need to put Mr. Avadian on mechanical soft food."

I panic. *Gulp! This is it! He's dying!* I take a deep breath to slow my racing heart. Sounding as calm as I can muster, "Yes, uhhh, mechanical soft. Why?"

"He's not eating his food."

"Why?"

"He's having difficulty swallowing."

I can see it now; the next step is a feeding tube! "Oh, he cannot swallow? Is this like pureed food?"

"No, our cook cuts up the food so Mr. Avadian can easily chew and then swallow it. Pureed food is the *next* step."

Silence.

"Hello?"

"Yes . . . this is the beginning of the end, isn't it?"

"No, Mr. Avadian is doing quite well. He just needs a little help to get his food down."

In February I answer the phone and hear: "This is [person's name] from the Antelope Valley Care Center. Mr. Avadian has pneumonia."

"How did he get it?"

"I'll have you talk with the nurse."

"Brenda, he has a fever. He caught an infection. The x-ray shows lower-lobe infiltrates," the nurse says.

Yeah, whatever those are! This is the end. I know it! I need to talk to someone about hospice.

"He's on oxygen right now. But he needs antibiotics."

I definitely need to talk to someone about hospice! Oxygen? This is the end. My frantic insides defy my outward composure, "Okay, give him antibiotics."

I write to June Kolf, a dear friend and former hospice volunteer coordinator and author of grief-related books. She asks, "Why are they giving him antibiotics? Brenda, did you know pneumonia is nicknamed *the old person's friend*?"

"No."

"Yes, it's called that because it often releases people from this life when other diseases cannot. Can I help *you*?"

"Uhhh . . . " June is sweet; my brain goes empty with her open invitation to help.

"Right now you probably need more care and support than your dad."

I keep her comment about pneumonia in mind for next time.

Mardig recovers. He seems to be constantly tired. Sometimes when David and I visit him, we can't get him to wake up. We visit other residents and then go home. He needs more and more rest these days.

Early March another call comes: "We need your approval to place your father in a geri-chair."

What? A geri-chair? It's hard enough seeing him in the wheelchair restrained by a posey! Now, you're telling me you want MY approval to place him in a geri-chair, like all the other residents lining the hallways, their mouths hanging open in a half-dead stupor? My mind races. Yet, like the earlier calls, I try to sound calm. "A geri-chair? Are you sure? Why?"

"Well, Mr. Avadian keeps falling out of his wheelchair. A CNA (certified nurse assistant) found him on the floor still strapped at the hip and to the wheelchair."

"Is he all right?"

"Yes, he has a little bruising on his arm and leg."

"But a geri-chair? Aren't there any other options? He'll become like the other residents in geri-chairs . . . you know . . . drooling with their mouths hanging open in a half-dead stupor, ignored in the hallways." *Did I just say that aloud?*

"Your dad is a lot more functional than some of our other residents. You don't have to worry about this. This is for his safety."

"But . . . "

"Next time you come in, talk with the director of nurses about this. For now, I need your approval."

I exhale a long SIGH. "Uhhh, okay."

Mardig looks more comfortable sitting in the geri-chair than in the wheelchair. Even the staff agrees. He sits in an upright position with a restraint. He appears content. I am happy, for the moment.

Just when things are going well, I receive another call. Mardig's heart rate is above 100. He's on oxygen. They are checking him for pneumonia . . . again.

I start asking questions about hospice.

(Below) Martin Avadian sits in a wheelchair, restrained by a posey to prevent him from falling. Despite David and Brenda's attempts to get him to laugh, on this day, Martin didn't seem to have any energy, not even for a smile. He looked preoccupied. This photo was taken on February 9, 2001, fifty days before he passed away. He would have been ninety-one years old.

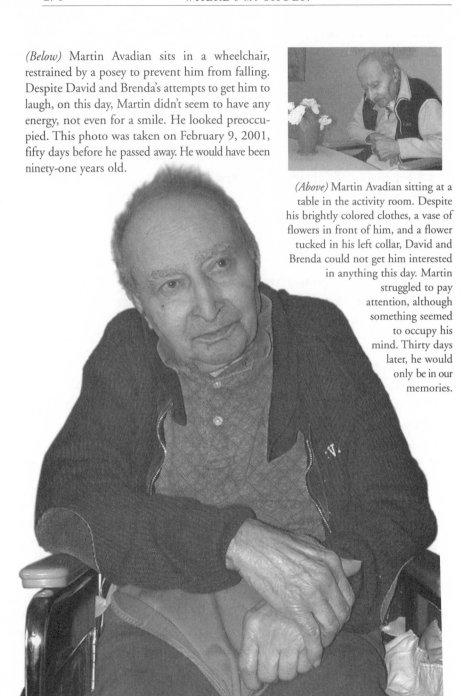

(Above) Martin Avadian sitting at a table in the activity room. Despite his brightly colored clothes, a vase of flowers in front of him, and a flower tucked in his left collar, David and Brenda could not get him interested in anything this day. Martin struggled to pay attention, although something seemed to occupy his mind. Thirty days later, he would only be in our memories.

CHAPTER 23

Mardig Makes
Life's Ultimate Transition

F riday morning, March 30, 2001. We try to finish feeding Mardig his breakfast. In the activity room, which doubles as an assisted feeding room, I sit at his side and David sits in front of him. I scoop warm cereal with a spoon and place it in Mardig's slightly open mouth. He chews the food a couple times and then closes his eyes. His head drops onto his chest. He appears to sleep. I don't want him to choke with food in his mouth, so I tickle his cheeks. He opens his eyes a crack, turns his lowered head against his chest, catches a glimpse of me, closes his eyes, and rotates his head back to rest.

I ask David to try, since he's sitting directly in front of him. The certified nurse assistant who was feeding Mardig when we arrived says residents cooperate more when they can see who's feeding them. She moved to help two other residents after we arrived. David tries. Again, my father opens his mouth, then his eyes, and takes the food. He chews several times, then closes his eyes, his head drops back onto his chest. David doesn't tolerate this behavior. He tickles my father's cheeks. When Mardig doesn't respond, David rubs his throat in order to get him to swallow. I laugh.

"What?" David asks, smiling. "Well, it worked for Mr. B!" he explains. *Mister B was the family dog during his childhood.*

"My father's not a dog," I say, laughing.

We don't know what to do. Here we are, two educated professionals, and we can't even feed a man in late-stage Alzheimer's. Then, it hits us. Since Mardig chews his food thoroughly before swallowing, maybe he'll wake up and start chewing if he feels his mouth is full. We take turns filling his mouth. His cheeks swell up like a chipmunk's.

Mardig does not move.

Now what are we going to do?

"We can't leave him this way. We have to remove the food!"

"How are we going to do that," David asks.

I put the empty spoon to my father's mouth. He doesn't react. I place a drinking straw between his lips. No response. David rubs the back of the spoon on Mardig's lips. Nothing.

Laughing at our predicament, we try to work together to part his lips and teeth in order to empty his mouth. Mardig opens his mouth. The food rests in his cheeks. David squeezes his cheeks as I try to spoon out the food.

"Brenda! What *are* you doing?"

I look up at the CNA who was feeding him when we walked in.

Feeling like a child who's in trouble, I look at her and try to defend myself. "We're trying to feed him and he keeps falling asleep!"

"No, no! My poor man," she says. "Mr. Avadian was eating nicely for me earlier!"

"Well, that's because you're a mom and you know how to feed people and make them swallow."

Shaking her head, "No. No. Poor Mr. Avadian."

Trying to get empathy for our situation, I add, "Obviously, I need lessons in feeding!"

We both laugh.

The CNAs and staff who work with my father know David's and my sense of humor, and feel comfortable teasing us.

"So, what are you trying to do to him now?"

"We're trying to empty his mouth because it's full and he's sleeping!"

"Do you want me to help?"

"Yes! That would be nice," I eagerly say and get up.

"No, it'll be easier from here."

David moves so she can sit in front of Mardig.

She says something to him and he opens his eyes slightly. She places the spoon to his lips, he focuses on her, his eyes open wide, and then starts chewing. He swallows the food and drinks his nutritional supplement through the straw.

"How'd you do that?" I ask, flabbergasted by how easily she fed him.

She laughs. "You just need to know how to feed him."

"Obviously! But seriously, how did you do that?"

"Some residents take their solid food easier with liquids. See? I give him a spoonful and then I offer him his drink."

"Hmmm, you have a special touch. Or maybe he likes the way you look!"

We laugh.

"Anyway, you'd better feed him from now on, or else he'll starve with us around!"

Earlier in March, I started asking about hospice care. As the grip of Alzheimer's tightened around Mardig's life, I knew the time was near when blood would stop coursing through his veins. I talked with the nurses at the AVCC, Mardig's doctor, June Kolf, the social worker at the Lancaster Adult Day Health Care Center, and friends who placed their loved ones on hospice. Those who worked closely with Mardig said hospice was a long way off. I didn't feel comfortable with their assessment, but resigned myself to use the time to finish other things. *I could be wrong.*

I still needed to revise the Advance Directives and had been telling the staff at the AVCC I planned to update them. After a while, they continued reminding me to update them. Among all the things I accomplished each week, I kept postponing this. Yet, with Mardig's continued decline I had to do it. He had two bouts of pneumonia and this was no way for a person with such diminished capacity to suffer. The Advance Directive on file instructed the staff to revive him and then take him to the hospital where doctors could assess his condition. We would consult with the doctors and then decide what type of medical care Mardig required, if any. Lately, however, I was telling the staff, if anything happens, let him go in peace.

I also told the staff, fellow caregivers, and friends, I wanted to be by Mardig's side as he passed away. To be certain I was near enough in the event Mardig's health declined rapidly, I turned down opportunities to travel overseas.

Dying doesn't have to be a lonely process. When my time comes, I'd like to be surrounded by family and friends. I may appear to be sedated, but at some level, I'll be aware of everyone's presence.

Saturday evening, March 31, David and I meet his co-worker and his wife for dinner at a local Mexican restaurant. We have not been out socially in a while and this is a welcome diversion. We bring our cell phones in case there's an urgent call. But once inside, the signals are weak. We've had these problems for over a year and became so frustrated we turn off both phones.

Nibbling on tortilla chips and hot and mild salsas, while sipping margaritas, David and his co-worker start talking about work. David had gotten a job at Lockheed Martin and was commuting a half-hour round trip each day instead of four hours. Even though I used to work at Lockheed and was familiar with their topic, work-related conversations during social outings are not my idea of fun. I start making funny faces and then David's co-worker's wife and I begin teasing them to have mercy on us and change the subject. Of course, they stop talking and then there's silence. For a moment, no one has anything to say. Thankfully, our meals arrive quickly and we eat the large portions without a care in the world. We split a dessert of fried ice cream, when David's co-worker and wife realize their children's baby-sitter is scheduled to leave at 9:30.

I enjoyed myself so much I could have stayed out all night.

David and I arrive home by 9:40 and listen to our messages. The first message left at 6:10 p.m. is from the AVCC. My father has suffered a massive stroke and is unconscious. I don't believe what I hear, so I play the message again.

"Mrs. Avadian? Brenda, Mr. Avadian had a seizure, then a massive stroke. Please call us. He is unconscious. We're trying to revive him. Please call us immediately."

The next message sounds more frantic.

"Brenda, we need to take your father to the hospital. We put him on oxygen. Please call. I know you said not to revive him . . . to let him go in peace, but we don't have it in writing. Please call us immediately."

In the background I hear a voice, "Call their cell phones and leave messages for them at work."

The third message: "Brenda? Brenda! Please call! We called the hospital and the ambulance is on its way to pick up Mr. Avadian. We have to do this per your written instructions in our files."

The next message is somber. "Brenda, your father did not go to the hospital. He passed away at 6:40 p.m. I'm so sorry."

The last message: "Brenda, we've been trying to reach you and David on your cell phones and at work. Please call us. We have your father in a private room if you'd like to see him. The mortuary is sending someone to pick him up at ten."

I breathe deeply. In less than ninety seconds, I have ridden a verbal roller coaster. A flurry of thoughts rushes through my mind. My now empty heart echoes as I try to grasp the emotions I am feeling. *My father is dead. He is no more. He is gone. I can't visit him anymore. David can't tease him and see how he responds.* Adrenaline flows quickly and my nerves are firing fast. David turns from the answering machine and looks at me. Despite what is happening inside me, externally I feel completely numb. *How can I be numb while my insides are churning?* I don't react. For the time being, I am frozen.

Then my sister's and my pledge flashes before me: If a major life-change occurs to anyone in our family, we will notify each other, even if we're not getting along. I call. It is after midnight in Wisconsin. As the answering machine plays her message, my mind flies in a million directions. I don't remember leaving a message.

David and I depart for the nursing home. I want to get there before my father is taken to the mortuary. I also want to talk with the staff to learn exactly what happened.

When we enter the building, the staff greets us warmly, with tear-filled eyes. They come forward, take my hands, and hold me while expressing their sorrows. Numb, yet focused on seeing my father, I hastily accept their sympathies as I make my way toward the private room where Mardig is laid to rest.

The lights are dim and the curtains are drawn for privacy. Two CNAs I've not met before are paying their respects. When they see David and I enter, they excuse themselves. It's late in the evening and the quiet is both reverential and eerie.

My father lies peacefully upon his deathbed, a sheet covers him except for his neck and head. A rolled up towel under his chin prevents his mouth from dropping open as his muscles release after death.

David and I walk to the opposite sides of the bed. My insides are still racing, and my heart feels hollow. I try to calm down, to embrace the quiet. Mardig has been released from all the indignities of late-stage Alzheimer's. He would not have wanted to live knowing some-one was helping him bathe, use the toilet, and cleaning him after-ward. He will no longer have to be fed like an infant, even though he enjoyed the attention.

I calm down as we stand in silence, each of us deep within our thoughts. I am sad, but feel no tears. He's been dying a little for so long. I've been grieving a long time. I think about how each of us deals with death.

"He's no longer in his body. Mardig sees everything now," David says softly. Born and raised Catholic, David believes my father is now at peace in heaven, released of this deadly Alzheimer's disease. "He understands everything now," David adds. *I wonder what it's like to see and understand everything.*

I was raised in a non-practicing Christian household. We were born Protestants. Our parents sent us to a small neighborhood Lutheran church. I don't know why, when there were other churches closer to home. All I remember was placing the offering in the collection basket each Sunday and how the Bible schoolteacher could not answer questions to my satisfaction.

"Where is heaven?" I'd ask, craning my neck to look out of the church basement windows.

"Above the clouds."

"How high above the clouds?"

"Way high."

"Well, where do the people stand?"

"Above the clouds."

"They can't stand above the clouds. They'd fall right through."

"They don't stand *on* the clouds."

"Well, how do angels sit on clouds?"

It went on and on. My need for facts didn't mesh with faith-based beliefs so, after several years and my parents' begrudging consent, I stopped attending.

Religion is a deeply personal belief and way of life; it can endear people to one another or alienate them. In this vein, I see myself as a spiritual person, who studies world religions.

With these thoughts in my mind, I gaze at my father. Whether or not he can see me, I want to be respectful of him, his body, and my memories of him. This man helped give me life forty-one years ago; even though he became the child I cared for at the end of his life. Am I *thinking* too much about his passing and not *feeling* enough, I wonder. Possibly. I accept that he is gone. In a way, I agree with David, he is out there. But he is also inside me. This is enough to comfort me.

I fix my attention on Mardig. I observe every nuance. His eyelids quiver. "David, look at his eyelids. Are they moving?"

"No, I didn't see that. I think I see a pulse in his neck."

"Look! He's breathing."

David watches my father's chest.

"I think we're trying to breathe life back into him."

David chuckles softly.

I ask David to help me cut a lock of Mardig's short hair. I wanted to do this, months earlier, but the time was never right. I can imagine Mardig laughing as I explain what I'm doing. I can almost hear him say, "Go ahead. If you can find some up there, it's yours."

I want to see his hands. There's something about a person's hands. I want to look at them one last time.

We carefully pull back the sheet. He's wearing a clean white T-shirt and his hands are folded above his abdomen. David and I stare at his hands for a long time. I rest my hand on top of his. His hands are no cooler than when he was alive. David rests his hand on Mardig's arm.

Suddenly there's a noise. Our moments of reverence and silence are interrupted by the man from the mortuary who has arrived to take *MY father*! We watch as he gathers up Mardig in the sheet, and with another man's help, places Mardig on the gurney. They tighten restraints around his body so he doesn't fall off as they wheel him out.

They travel down the hallway, out the back doors, to a van with no windows. We watch a while longer until they drive away.

David and I walk back inside to talk with the nurse. She explains they tried to give Mardig oxygen and, when he did not respond, they tried CPR, but he had slipped away. She assures us Mardig did not suffer nor did he feel pain. I am relieved. Mardig said he wanted to die in his sleep. In a way, he did.

We leave the facility just before eleven.

I call my sister. I hoped, at 1:10 a.m. her time, she might answer the phone thinking it was an emergency. Disappointed, I leave a message on her answering machine.

Next, I phone my brother and hear a woman's voice answer. Not thinking clearly, I think it's his girlfriend. A moment later, I realize it's his answering service. *What should I say? How do I let him know what happened? This is an answering service! I can't leave a message like this!*

"Is there a message?" she asks.

"Yes, please tell [my brother] his father died this evening at 6:40 p.m. California time and that he can call his sister, Brenda, at . . . " I leave my home phone number and area code.

As David and I calm down after a whirlwind evening, I hope what a few caregivers told me turns out to be true: "After your father's gone, there will be no one left in your immediate family; so, your sister, brother, and you will grow closer."

Each time the phone rings, I hope it's my sister or brother. Each time I go online to check my e-mails, I hope to read one of theirs.

The following day, which is also the eighth anniversary of my mother's passing, we rest and reminisce. We call Mardig's two brothers, other relatives, David's family, and friends.

Monday arrives. I start working before 6:00 a.m. There is much to do. I am finishing the first volume of the *Finding the JOY* book series and gathering stories for the second volume. *How can there be JOY in Alzheimer's when Alzheimer's took my father?* I have to follow-up on the administrative details after Mardig's passing. *Let's see, I need to contact two attorneys, the accountant, the trust administrator, our other family members, and, oh, I have to get a death certificate.*

Meanwhile, there are more phone calls and e-mails. Friends, colleagues, and caregivers ask, "Will you continue this work?" "Will you keep writing books and helping families?" "Will you still talk about your experience?" *Wow! I'd better give this some serious thought! It's going to be hard now, because my father's no longer living. Anything I say will be borne out of past experience; no more current stories to share.*

On Tuesday morning, I juggle talking on the phone, replying to e-mails, and taking care of the legal obligations after someone dies. I tell everyone Mardig's memorial tribute will occur sometime between Friday and Sunday.

Eight years earlier, when my mother died, I wanted to have a memorial service with my family. I witnessed Mardig's sadness when my brother and sister did not join us. Without them involved, Mardig and I lost the desire to do anything. Harboring this regret for eight years, I vowed to have a memorial for my father. Mardig's walk through Alzheimer's had a significant impact on David's and my lives. Equally important, his journey touched people beyond our immediate circle of caregivers, friends, relatives, and colleagues. Readers and listeners of the first edition of *"Where's my shoes?"* and audiences around the country walked this road with us. They feel a part of our family and comment on how their journey parallels ours. We have to honor this. My father's walk touched us all.

Now, if I could only find a place for his memorial tribute.

In the afternoon, I put everything aside to do something for me. I attend a support group at the adult day care center regularly. These caregivers have become my family and I want to be with them. I even participate in an on-line chat in the evening with caregivers from around the world.

Wednesday arrives and we still don't have a place for the tribute. This is harder than I expect. I feel overwhelmed trying to plan the event, notify everyone, not forget someone, create an invitation, etc. *When do I fit in time for grieving?*

Caregivers volunteer to help find a place where people can freely share their memories, eat, and spend time together.

David and I must also squeeze in time to finalize our tax return, due in less than two weeks.

What a mess, all this paperwork and coordination!

More phone calls and e-mails pour in from friends, distant relatives, and colleagues from around the world. These are followed by letters and cards. More people offer to help. I especially treasure the cards and e-mails from those who write a special message. Mardig's attorney sends passages from the Talmud mixed with his feelings of loss.

June Kolf, whose husband succumbed to cancer, writes: *You can both feel good about the way you handled the difficult situation and the way you used Martin's disease to help others. Your book will live on, giving your dad a unique kind of immortality.*

Diane Blake, caregiver to her mother, writes: *As part of the "sisterhood of Alzheimer's daughters," I know that you "lost" your father, as you knew him, a long time ago. I also know that you would have wanted to be with him in his final "physical" passing, but I am sure that you are grateful he passed so quickly and painlessly, for his sake.*

He has left so much of himself with you—his intellect, his sense of humor, his work ethic.

My heart goes out to you "dear girl" knowing the challenges that lie ahead in the coming weeks and months. You are fortunate to have David by your side, to help add ballast in your decisions.

A colleague and dear friend, Jill Wilson, paints a hopeful picture of the stars: *When my dad died, one of my dear friends gave me a card that read "Perhaps they are not the stars, but rather openings in Heaven where the love of our lost ones shines down to let us know they are with us." When I look up on a starry night, I always feel much better.*

You'll miss him. I miss my dad, but how lucky you are to have your written memories right there at your side. You've shared them with so many. We do mourn with you.

A fellow caregiver's e-mail expresses many people's reactions: *I loved Martin . . . he was so cute and feisty. He brought joy and smiles to all of us who were privileged to know him for a little while.*

Among the hundreds of messages that arrived from around the world, not a single card, e-mail, or telephone call is from my brother or sister. I feel sad, hurt, and angry.

Thursday, per his wish, my father is cremated in Glendale. I feel awkward about this, because his body will be reduced to ashes.

His cremains are returned to the funeral home on Friday where I pick them up. The crematory included a certificate so I can take my father's ashes to Milwaukee. Until then, I place the box of his cremains in my home office and continue working. I am surprised my father's physical being has been reduced to this small box.

One week after Mardig died, on the afternoon of April 7, we gather for a memorial tribute at a hall in a nearby Lutheran Church. The location turned out to be notable in two ways. First, Mardig enjoyed going to adult day care in this same complex. Second, our parents attended a Lutheran church; perhaps, this was a way of closing that chapter by celebrating his life in one.

Given Mardig's widespread impact and the joy he brought to those in his life, we decided to have a "Celebration of Life." The new owner, management team, and staff from the Antelope Valley Care Center came. They played music, sang, and prayed. Relatives, care-givers, friends, and colleagues attended. The local television and print media even paid tribute to Mardig.

Yet, there was a void. Two people were missing. Guests asked, "Are they here?" I looked around. My sister and brother never called nor showed. I tried not to dwell on who was *missing*. There were over eighty people HERE! We shared memories of Mardig and enjoyed a buffet of homemade multi-ethnic foods. What a touching tribute and truly a Celebration of Life!

CHAPTER 24

Mardig Lives On

F ollowing the memorial tribute, I looked forward to resting and reflecting; especially after the whirlwind of the last several years. Alas, there was no time. I had speaking engagements in seven cities.

How am I going to talk about my father in the past tense? It doesn't feel right. My days as a caregiver have ended. I won't have any new experiences to talk about. Anything I say will be in hindsight. What can I say to let family caregivers and professionals know I still walk in caregiver's shoes?

I considered returning to leadership and communications consulting; this time with a focus on healthcare. *Mardig is gone. What else could I possibly say?*

I gave the first speech. The audience rose and gave me a standing ovation. I nearly cried. With each subsequent speech, audiences responded more enthusiastically. Each time I told this story, I was honoring my father. Unexpectedly, I was also dealing with my loss.

In late May, I carried my father's cremains onto a plane. I had a business trip in Chicago. I looked down and silently talked to him.

After a long life, this is it, huh Mardig? Your third plane flight, and you're in my carry-on bag under the seat in front. Hmmm.

I set aside a day to drive up to Milwaukee to place his cremains next to my mother's. Accompanied by my aunt and uncle, I drove north to Milwaukee. We met Marva, my friend from college and the mother of David's and my godchildren. We held a mini memorial before ceremoniously placing his and my mother's cremains side by side (Marva's idea) in a golden urn. My uncle, who fought in World War II and has been living with Parkinson's disease for nearly a quarter-century, cried. His older brother, who he respected so much, was gone. I carried the urn back to the indoor niche my father had selected for my mother and himself. I was overcome by a deep sense of gratitude as I carried my parents' cremains, the two people who brought me into this world. I nearly lost my balance on the ladder as I placed the heavy urn on the shelf for display behind the glass.

We moved forward with our first title in the ground-breaking *Finding the JOY* series, *Finding the JOY in Alzheimer's: Caregivers Share the JOYFUL Times*.

The first Father's Day without Mardig was not as painful as the first Mother's Day after my mother's passing. In April 1993, while looking for a birthday card for my sister, I noticed all the Mother's Day cards. *I no longer have a mother!* My eyes welled up with tears and I fought to catch my breath. Even though David's parents are still alive, they are young and more like a brother and sister. I call them by their first names, Paul and Judi.

Sometimes I feel like an orphan. I have no immediate family members with whom to share my childhood. Overall, though, I am fortunate. I have partially filled this emptiness with new and rediscovered family members. Sally continues to fill the void left by my mother's passing, comforting me when I'm down, giving me encouragement when I need it, and talking sense into me when I don't make any. I am closer to my cousins, uncles, and aunts on my father's side and to more distant cousins on my mother's side. One of David's colleagues, Michael, has come into our lives. With his unique talent for bringing together strangers and turning them into friends, we now have become a family, always ready to help one another.

Nearly six months after my father died, I finally accepted Patti's repeated invitations to attend her bereavement group. Her husband, Ralph, passed away and she had been attending for about a year. I was so busy; I hadn't started to grieve. *Or had I? Maybe my speaking and writing was my way of working through my grief.* Attendees sat in a circle, introduced themselves, and talked about their loved ones. Men and women cried as they told their stories. Others laughed as they recalled happy memories. In fact, my first meeting was filled with more laughter than tears. At the end, I said, "This is the most fun I've had in a long time! And this is a bereavement group!"

Over the months, I learned to laugh more and gained an appreciation for different ways of grieving, all normal. Some people hold onto sentimental reminders of their loved one, while others discard everything, including selling their home. Some have their loved ones cremated, others have them embalmed and buried. Some keep their loved one's remains at home or in a niche, while others scatter the ashes in a special place. Some overcome their grief after several months, while others grieve the loss for a lifetime. Some form relations with special people and begin a new life of living together, while others enjoy a solo life of focused reflection.

Most importantly, I grew to accept my sister and brother. I became more comfortable with the idea of *not* having to understand their behavior. I stopped asking, "Why?" After calling, e-mailing, and sending them faxes, I live with their choice not to communicate.

It's been nearly four years and I still attend the bereavement group meetings. I've been attending the support group at the Lancaster Adult Day Health Care Center for over eight years. We share such personal details about our lives; we are more like a family than strangers brought together by a common need. It's hard to walk away from such a bond. And even though many of the original members have either passed on or are unable to attend, there are a few of us old-timers who return to the caregiving support group. Many of the deceased caregivers played an important role while I cared for my father. I share their stories when I speak.

If it weren't for my father's journey, I doubt I would feel such a strong sense of community.

For many months after Mardig's passing, when the details piled up and there was too much, or when I was in a hurry and everything seemed to be going wrong, I'd hear my father's words: "Keep your head about you!" It was his way of telling me to take a breath and concentrate on what I was doing so I would not get into an accident, make a mistake, or hurt myself. His words still guide me through the tough times. Sometimes I hear my mother's words more clearly, and I whine in self-pity. *Eem klookh-us beedie pai-tee!* (My head is going to explode!)

Even little things can seem overwhelming, like when Mardig received two requests for jury duty. I sent back the form with a note that he died. A second notice arrived; this time they required a doctor's note to attest to Mardig's inability to serve. This posed a bit of a challenge. I returned the form with a note: "We regret we are unable to find a doctor willing to declare Martin Avadian's inability to serve since he died." *SIGH, the price of bureaucracy!* At least we had a good laugh!

It took a year to finalize everything and to distribute what was left in the estate. The stock market bubble burst and with it, people's investments. Mardig's investments were impacted, but not to a large degree. Much of his estate went toward his care, which exceeded $300,000. A sizable amount went toward taxes. What remained was divided among us.

For nearly two years after he died, when I drove near the AVCC, I felt a strong urge to see Mardig. I still visit the residents and talk with family members. If I can help one resident smile or feel she'll be all right, I will have made a significant contribution. *Some day, that resident could be me!*

After the legal challenges and dreaded paperwork for my father's estate, David and I devoted two years to completing our living wills and estate plan. It took us this long, because we didn't want to do it. Each time we sat down to work on our will, we experienced headaches, neck aches, backaches, or imaginary excuses—anything, so as not to face these difficult choices. We are in our mid-forties, and according to some, we have completed our plans early. We hired the attorney who selflessly advised us and then referred us to a more qualified attorney when we were struggling to resolve key issues around my father's affairs. Despite the cost, getting our plan together will ensure our wishes are carried out the way we intend.

In 2004, we moved to a home on five acres of private land tucked within the Angeles National Forest. David reminds me my parents were looking for something similar when they looked for homes in California. Perhaps they're guiding us. As David and I settle in, we look forward to many years of happiness in this home with our friends and family—before we need long-term care.

To this day, my sister, brother, and I have not communicated. Looking through the photos of those days in April 1997, when we cleared out our father's home together, I remember the fun we had. I would love to see them again, to laugh, tease, and share memories of our childhood. I miss them.

Until then, I find balance with my ever-growing circle of friends and rediscovered extended family. I also know each time someone reads one of my books, contacts me, or invites me to speak, my father's memory stays alive. Mardig would be surprised and humbled knowing the last years of his life are helping so many. As worldwide awareness of the impact of this disease increases, I grow more confident that one day, when I'm sitting in a nursing home and I reach out for help, someone will approach and extend their hand to comfort me.

Thank you for letting us take this journey with you, Mardig.

Your memory lives on.

Appendix A

Tips for Caregivers

1. Learn about your loved one's disease so you know what to expect. For example, break tasks down into single easy-to-manage steps. Answer repeated questions as if each is the first time it was asked. Your loved one does not remember asking the question before.

2. Attend support group meetings in person or online. Ask questions, even if you think you know the answer. You're not alone. Others are walking the same road; together you can help one another.

3. Make direct eye contact and address your loved one where she is. If she is happy, smile and greet her enthusiastically. If he looks solemn, speak to him in a lower and more peaceful tone. Touch him and give him a hug, if appropriate.

4. It's okay to get frustrated and even angry. Find an appropriate outlet for your feelings, though. Try to get physical exercise or phone a fellow caregiver. At the very least, STOP and take a deep breath.

5. LAUGH. Find the JOY in the smallest things. SMILE.

6. Seek respite, even for five minutes. Martyrs are not heroes. NEVER say NEVER. Consider your options—adult day care,

in-home care, board and care, assisted living, skilled nursing facility.

7. Seek competent professional advice regarding legal, financial, and healthcare matters. Talk with someone you trust about the advice you receive. Have all your questions answered before you sign anything.

8. Most importantly, treat your loved one the way you want to be treated once you require care.

Ten Warning Signs of Alzheimer's

- ◆ Memory loss.

- ◆ Difficulty performing familiar tasks, such as preparing a meal, using a household appliance, or engaging in a hobby.

- ◆ Problems with language; for example, trying to find the right word to express a common item such as a hairbrush, comb, or key.

- ◆ Disorientation to time and place. Examples may include not knowing the year, time of day, or how to return home.

- ◆ Poor or decreased judgment as evidenced by giving large sums of money to solicitors, wearing inappropriate clothing for the weather (winter coat in the summer).

- ◆ Problems with abstract thinking, such as balancing a checkbook.

- ◆ Placing things in unusual places, i.e., a spoon is put in the toaster or the peanut butter is stored under the kitchen sink with the household cleaning supplies.

◆ Changes in mood or behavior.

◆ Noticeable changes in personality, including confusion, paranoia, or fear.

◆ Loss of initiative. Examples include sitting idle, watching television for hours at a time, excessive sleeping.

Material adapted with permission from the Alzheimer's Association Website: www.alz.org

For More Information . . .

ALZHEIMER'S ASSOCIATION
World leader in Alzheimer's research and support. Founded in 1980, this nationwide network of chapters offers support to individuals affected by Alzheimer's with 24/7 information and referral, safety services, and education and support groups.
225 North Michigan Ave. 17th Floor
Chicago, IL 60611-7633 U.S.A.
Tel. 800-272-3900 Website: www.alz.org

ALZHEIMER'S DISEASE EDUCATION AND REFERRAL (ADEAR)
Information about Alzheimer's disease and related disorders, a service of the National Institute on Aging (NIA).
P.O. Box 8250, Silver Spring, MD 20907-8250 U.S.A.
Tel: 800-438-4380 Website: www.alzheimers.org

ALZHEIMER'S DISEASE INTERNATIONAL
Umbrella organization of Alzheimer's associations around the world, which offer support and information to people with dementia and their caregivers.
45-46 Lower Marsh London SE1 7RG U.K.
Tel: +44-20-7620-3011 Website: www.alz.co.uk

AMERICAN SOCIETY ON AGING (ASA)
The largest professional membership association committed to enhancing the knowledge and skills of those working with older adults and their families. Founded in 1954.
833 Market St., Suite 511, San Francisco, CA 94103 U.S.A.
Tel: 415-974-9600 Toll-free: 800-537-9728
Website: www.asaging.org

THECAREGIVERSVOICE.COM
Gives a voice to the millions of caregivers who care for their loved ones. Access this site for news updates, links to other informative sites, and to submit your stories for the Finding the JOY series of books.
P.O. Box 589, Pearblossom, CA 93553-0589 U.S.A.
Tel: 661-944-1130 Website: www.TheCaregiversVoice.com

CLINICALTRIALS.GOV
Current information for locating federally and privately supported clinical trials for a wide range of diseases and conditions. Studies listed in the database are conducted primarily in all 50 of the United States and in over 90 countries.
Website: www.clinicaltrials.gov

DEMENTIA ADVOCACY AND SUPPORT NETWORK INTERNATIONAL (DASNI)
A worldwide organization by and for those with dementia, working together to improve quality of life.
P.O. Box 1645 Mariposa, California 95338 U.S.A.
Website: www.dasninternational.org

ELDERCARE LOCATOR
A free nationwide directory assistance service to help older persons and caregivers locate local support resources. Administered through the National Association of Area Agencies on Aging in Washington, D.C.
Tel: 800-677-1116
From outside the U.S.A. dial Spherix at 301-419-3900 and ask for the Eldercare Locator line.
Website: www.eldercare.gov

HOSPICE FOUNDATION OF AMERICA
Not-for-profit organization that provides leadership in the development and application of hospice and its philosophy of care. Through programs of professional development, research, public education, and information, assists those who cope personally or professionally with terminal illness, death, and the process of grief.
Website: www.hospicefoundation.org

NATIONAL ACADEMY OF ELDER LAW ATTORNEYS (NAELA)
Non-profit association assisting lawyers, bar organizations, and others working with older clients and their families. Established in 1987.
1604 N. Country Club Road Tucson, AZ 85716 U.S.A.
Tel: 520-881-4005 Website: www.naela.com

NATIONAL ADULT DAY SERVICES ASSOCIATION (NADSA)
The leading voice of the rapidly growing adult day service industry in the United States, and the national focal point for adult day service providers committed to providing its members with effective national advocacy, educational and networking opportunities, technical assistance, and research and communication services.
722 Grant Street, Suite L Herndon, Virginia 20170 U.S.A.
Tel: 703-435-8630 Toll-free: 800-558-5301
Website: www.nadsa.org

NATIONAL ALLIANCE FOR CAREGIVING
A coalition of 40 national organizations that conducts research and policy analysis, develops national programs, and works to increase public awareness of family caregiving issues across the life span.
4720 Montgomery Lane, 5th Floor, Bethesda, MD 20814
Website: www.caregiving.org E-mail: info@caregiving.org

NATIONAL ASSOCIATION OF PROFESSIONAL GERIATRIC CARE MANAGERS (GCM)
Professional organization of practitioners whose goal is the advancement of dignified care for the elderly and their families.
1604 N. Country Club Road, Tucson, AZ 85716-3102 U.S.A.
Tel: 520-881-8008 Website: www.caremanager.org

NATIONAL FAMILY CAREGIVERS ASSOCIATION (NFCA)
Grassroots organization created to educate, support, empower, and speak up for the millions of Americans who care for chronically ill, aged, or disabled loved ones. Inquire about free membership for family caregivers.
10400 Connecticut Avenue, Suite 500, Kensington, MD 20895-3944 U.S.A.
Tel: 301-942-6430 Toll-free: 800-896-3650
Website: www.nfcacares.org

NATIONAL HOSPICE AND PALLIATIVE CARE ORGANIZATION (NHPCO)
Founded in 1978, the oldest and largest nonprofit membership organization representing hospice and palliative care programs and professionals. Committed to improving end-of-life care and expanding access to hospice care to enhance the quality of life for people dying in America and their loved ones.
1700 Diagonal Road, Suite 625 Alexandria, Virginia 22314 U.S.A.
Tel: 703-837-1500 Website: www.nhpco.org

THERIBBON.COM
Free on-line newsletter for families and caregivers dealing with Alzheimer's disease and other dementias. Includes nightly chat for caregivers at www.theribbon.com/gatherplace
Website: www.theribbon.com

SAFE RETURN™ PROGRAM
Alzheimer's Association's nationwide program assisting in the identification, and safe and timely return of people with Alzheimer's disease and related disorders who wander. See "Alzheimer's Association" for more information.

Bibliography

Allen, Mary Emma. *When we Become the Parent to our Parents*.
Plymouth: MEA Productions, 1998.

Avadian, Brenda, MA, ed. *Finding the JOY in Alzheimer's: Caregivers Share the Joyful Times*. Lancaster: North Star Books, 2002.

Avadian, Brenda, MA, ed. *Finding the JOY in Alzheimer's~Vol. 2: When Tears are Dried with Laughter*. Lancaster: North Star Books, 2003.

Avadian, Brenda, MA. *"Where's my shoes?" My Father's Walk Through Alzheimer's*. (1st ed.) Unabridged Audio narrated by Barbara Caruso, Prince Frederick: Recorded Books, 2000.

Bell, Virginia and Troxel, David, MPHS. *The Best Friends Approach to Alzheimer's Care*. Baltimore: Health Professions Press, 2003.

Brackey, Jolene. *Creating Moments of JOY for the Person with Alzheimer's or Dementia: A Journal for Caregivers*. West Lafayette: Purdue University Press, 2000.

Cohen, Elizabeth. *The House on Beartown Road: A Memoir of Learning and Forgetting*. New York: Random House, 2003

DeBaggio, Thomas. *Losing my Mind: An Intimate Look at Life with Alzheimer's*. New York: Free Press, 2002.

Ewing, Wayne. *Tears in God's Bottle: Reflections on Alzheimer's Caregiving*. Tuscon: WhiteStone Circle Press, 1999.

Feil, Naomi. *The Validation Breakthrough: Simple Techniques for Communicating with People with "Alzheimer's-Type Dementia"* (2nd ed.). Baltimore: Health Professions Press, 2002.

FitzRay, B.J. *Alzheimer's Activities: Hundreds of Activities for Men and Women with Alzheimer's Disease and Related Disorders*. Windsor: Rayve Productions, 2001

Glass, Sue and W. Yunker, illus. *Remember Me?: Alzheimer's Through the Eyes of a Child*. Green Bay: Raven Tree Press, 2003.

Gruetzner, Howard. *Alzheimer's: A Caregiver's Guide and Sourcebook* (3rd ed.). New York: John Wiley & Sons, 2001.

Kolf, June Cerza. *Comfort & Care in a Final Illness*. Tucson: Fisher Books, 1999.

Kolf, June Cerza. *How Can I Help?* Tucson: Fisher Books, 1999.

Lokvig, Jytte, MA and Becker, John D., MD. *Alzheimer's A to Z: A Quick Reference Guide*. Oakland: New Harbinger Publications, Inc., 2004.

Mace, Nancy L., MA and Peter V. Rabins, MD, MPH. *The 36-Hour Day: A Family Guide to Caring for Persons with Alzheimer Disease, Related Dementing Illnesses, and Memory Loss in Later Life.* (Revised Edition). New York: Warner Books, 2001

McLeod, Beth Witrogen, ed. *And Thou Shalt Honor: The Caregiver's Companion*. Emmaus: Rodale, 2002.

Meyer, Maria with Derr, Paula. *The Comfort of Home: An illustrated Step-by-Step Guide for Caregivers*. Portland: CareTrust Publications, 1998.

Peterson, Betsy. *Voices of Alzheimer's: Courage, Humor, Hope, and Love in the Face of Dementia*. Cambridge: DeCapo Press, 2004.

Peterson, Ronald, MD, PhD, ed. *Mayo Clinic on Alzheimer's Disease*. Rochester: Mayo Clinic Health Information, 2002.

Sarnoff, Schiff, Harriet. *How Did I Become My Parent's Parent?* New York: Viking Press, 1996.

Shenk, David. *The Forgetting. Alzheimer's: A Portrait of an Epidemic*. New York: Anchor, 2003.

Shriver, Maria. *What's Happening to Grandpa?* New York: Little Brown & Company, 2004.

Snyder, Lisa, LCSW. *Speaking Our Minds: Personal Reflections from Individuals with Alzheimer's*. New York: W.H. Freeman and Company, 2000.

INDEX

ORDER INFORMATION

Ask for the fully revised and expanded *second* edition of
"Where's my shoes?"
at your neighborhood bookstore or library
or
Order through any online retailer.

Help support groups and organizations that help people
with Alzheimer's and their families when you
ORDER TOLL FREE 1-800-852-4890
(Credit card orders only)
or
Order through our Website
http://www.TheCaregiversVoice.com/books

Also check out our
Finding the JOY in Alzheimer's series of books,
offering stories, poems, and photos of hope and joy.

We welcome your comments.

Write to the author at
BrendaAvadian@TheCaregiversVoice.com

NORTH STAR BOOKS
P. O. Box 589
Pearblossom, CA • 93553-0589 • U.S.A.
Tel: 661.944.1130
E-mail: NorthStarBooks@avradionet.com